SAFETY AND RISK IN SOCIETY

INVESTIGATING PATIENT SAFETY

SAFETY AND RISK IN SOCIETY

Additional books and e-books in this series can be found on Nova's website under the Series tab.

SAFETY AND RISK IN SOCIETY

INVESTIGATING PATIENT SAFETY

GLORIA HALE
EDITOR

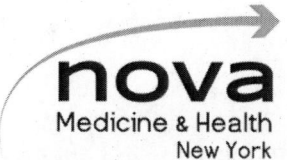

Copyright © 2020 by Nova Science Publishers, Inc.

All rights reserved. No part of this book may be reproduced, stored in a retrieval system or transmitted in any form or by any means: electronic, electrostatic, magnetic, tape, mechanical photocopying, recording or otherwise without the written permission of the Publisher.

We have partnered with Copyright Clearance Center to make it easy for you to obtain permissions to reuse content from this publication. Simply navigate to this publication's page on Nova's website and locate the "Get Permission" button below the title description. This button is linked directly to the title's permission page on copyright.com. Alternatively, you can visit copyright.com and search by title, ISBN, or ISSN.

For further questions about using the service on copyright.com, please contact:
Copyright Clearance Center
Phone: +1-(978) 750-8400   Fax: +1-(978) 750-4470   E-mail: info@copyright.com

NOTICE TO THE READER

The Publisher has taken reasonable care in the preparation of this book, but makes no expressed or implied warranty of any kind and assumes no responsibility for any errors or omissions. No liability is assumed for incidental or consequential damages in connection with or arising out of information contained in this book. The Publisher shall not be liable for any special, consequential, or exemplary damages resulting, in whole or in part, from the readers' use of, or reliance upon, this material. Any parts of this book based on government reports are so indicated and copyright is claimed for those parts to the extent applicable to compilations of such works.

Independent verification should be sought for any data, advice or recommendations contained in this book. In addition, no responsibility is assumed by the Publisher for any injury and/or damage to persons or property arising from any methods, products, instructions, ideas or otherwise contained in this publication.

This publication is designed to provide accurate and authoritative information with regard to the subject matter covered herein. It is sold with the clear understanding that the Publisher is not engaged in rendering legal or any other professional services. If legal or any other expert assistance is required, the services of a competent person should be sought. FROM A DECLARATION OF PARTICIPANTS JOINTLY ADOPTED BY A COMMITTEE OF THE AMERICAN BAR ASSOCIATION AND A COMMITTEE OF PUBLISHERS.

Additional color graphics may be available in the e-book version of this book.

Library of Congress Cataloging-in-Publication Data

Names: Hale, Gloria, editor.
Title: Investigating patient safety / [edited by] Gloria Hale.
Description: New York : Nova Science Publishers, Inc., [2020] | Series:
  Safety and Risk in Society | Includes bibliographical references
  and index. |
Identifiers: LCCN 2020000116 (print) | LCCN 2020000117 (ebook) | ISBN
  9781536173444 (paperback) | ISBN 9781536173451 (adobe pdf)
Subjects: LCSH: Medical errors--Prevention. | Patients--Safety measures. |
  Investigations.
Classification: LCC R729.8 .I58 2020 (print) | LCC R729.8 (ebook) | DDC
  610.28/9--dc23
LC record available at https://lccn.loc.gov/2020000116
LC ebook record available at https://lccn.loc.gov/2020000117

Published by Nova Science Publishers, Inc. † New York

CONTENTS

Preface		vii
Chapter 1	The Error as a Parameter of Healthcare Quality *Vasiliki Kapaki*	1
Chapter 2	Pursuing Patient Safety through Researching and Reducing Diagnostic Errors and Applying a Systematic Approach to Diagnosis *Ami Schattner*	29
Chapter 3	The Implementation of the Common Assessment Framework in Public Healthcare Organizations: Improving Patient Safety through Improvement of Organizational Performance *Stella Korouli, Vasiliki Kapaki and Adamantia Englezopoulou*	71
Chapter 4	Patient Safety without Patient Advocacy is Improbable, as They are Synonymous: Is There a Theory-Practice-Ethics Gap? *Manfred Mortell*	97

Chapter 5	Air Embolism and Hypothermia Associated with Intravenous Fluid Therapy: Risk Management Considerations *Nickolas A. MacDougall and Mark E. Comunale*	**121**
Index		**145**
Related Nova Publications		**151**

PREFACE

Investigating Patient Safety opens with a summary on the main theories representative of human error, such as: "Bad Apples Theory", "Normal Accident Theories" and "High Reliability Organizations Theory".

Following this, the authors define mistakes in the diagnostic process, identifying their major causes and suggesting several principles for optimal, bias-free diagnoses.

Evidence is presented which supports the idea that the Common Assessment Framework is a total quality management tool that public organizations can use for free for their self-assessment, aiming to improving their administrative capacity and services without having to ask for support from external sources.

An analytical exploration of patient advocacy related to patient safety and the concept of a "Theory-Practice-Ethics gap" is presented, reinforcing the importance of their synonymous relationship for trustworthy healthcare practices.

The concluding chapter proposes that inline fluid warming devices must employ the safest technology to ensure patients are not exposed to additional risks during the active warming of infused fluids.

Chapter 1 - Human error is a term that is often referred to the case of an accident, whether it concerns the workplace or not. It is often used as a "causal umbrella" to easily explain an accident. The rendering of human error is preceded by the deficiencies in the system, but without necessarily incriminating the victim, since human error is considered to be a natural (albeit unpredictable) outcome of human functions, as was done previously by invoking metaphysical causes (Acts of God). So the study of human error in some cases accepted the criticism that exists to serve this purpose. Usually the "finger" shows workers and victims of accidents as the problem and therefore the most appropriate study subject as they are the ones most involved.

Indeed, the accident is the result of many interacting factors (people, materials, processes) and the attribution of causality to only one of them is an incomplete process, since taking the appropriate measures to others can be avoided. Human error cannot be independent of the system that is occurring, nor is it the only cause of an accident.

However, this does not mean that human error does not exist or is not a causal factor of accidents that should be studied. Unless the potential involuntary actions of an individual are studied, it is not possible to design the means and procedures that will prevent these actions from evolving into accidents.

The study of human error is mainly based on the science of Psychology and Mechanics and less on the Principles of Operations Research. In the chapter are summarized the main representative theories of human error such as Bad Apples Theory, Normal Accident Theories and High Reliability Organizations Theory etc.

Chapter 2 - Adverse patient outcomes, including mortality, are often associated with iatrogenic harm. While medication errors, health care-associated infections and falls have long been the focus of attention and a well-established target of intervention, diagnostic errors have been relatively neglected. Nevertheless, errors in diagnosis (including incorrect, missed or delayed diagnosis) constitute an important facet of patient safety, and may also be preventable.

In contrast with the prevailing view that advances in scientific knowledge and technology have practically eliminated the possibility of errors in diagnosis, data from autopsy studies, readmissions research and claims data reveal that these errors continue to occur with an estimated incidence of 10-20% and not infrequently, dire consequences. Therefore, further study is required to illuminate the multifactorial origins of diagnostic errors and develop techniques for improving clinical reasoning and the diagnostic process thereby reducing unwanted errors.

The authors define mistakes in the diagnostic process, identify their major causes, and suggest several principles of optimal, bias-free diagnosis based on the SOAP mnemonic stressing a Systematic methodical approach, Observation and listening to the patient, Accessing databases for patient-tailored decisions, and adopting a Personal, humanistic, patient-centered communication to reduce diagnostic errors and enhance patient safety.

Chapter 3 - The Common Assessment Framework (CAF) constitutes a holistic analysis of the performance of one organization, approaching it from different perspectives simultaneously. According to this, the excellent results for the organizational performance, citizens/customers and society rely on leadership, planning/design, human resources, partnerships, resources, as well as administrative processes. CAF is based on 8 basic principles, the so called "Excellence Principles", namely Results orientation, Focus on citizen/customer, Leadership and Consistency of aim, Management through processes and facts, Development and participation of human resources, Continuous learning, Innovation and improvement, Development of partnerships and Corporate social responsibility. These principles have been incorporated in the CAF structure through 9 criteria, which are further analyzed in 28 subcriteria. Each of the principles has 4 maturity levels, which define over time the course of one organization towards excellence. The CAF 9 criteria represent the main aspects that need to be taken into consideration during the analysis of any organization. These are categorized in 5 criteria- enablers, which cover what the organization does (Leadership, Strategy & Planning, Human Resources, Partnerships & Resources and Processes) and 4 criteria- results, which cover what the organization achieves (Citizens/Customers oriented results, Human Resources oriented results, Society oriented results and Key performance results). By conducting a self-assessment Public Organizations may define in their function their strengths, as well as areas for improvement. The self-assessment process is guided by a specific rating system. The CAF implementation is a continuous process, as the conclusions from one assessment should lead to a plan with improvement actions, which, after their implementaion, should be re-assessed using the CAF, so to achieve continuous administrative improvement. As a conclusion, the CAF is a Total Quality Management (TQM) tool that Public Organizations can use for free for their self-assessment, aiming at improving their administrative capacity and services, without having to ask for support from external sources.

Chapter 4 - The aim of a culture of safety in healthcare is to reduce and/or eliminate the risk of harm to patients. However, despite a universal stance towards patient safety, since the Institute of Medicine's landmark report of 2000, *"To Err is Human, building a safer health system"* there remains a disturbing escalation in the healthcare errors among hospitalized patients. This underscores trepidations about healthcare professionals and providers'aptitude as effective and caring patient advocates to provide high quality, safe care. In the context of these healthcare mistakes, the *"Theory-Practice gap"* is often cited as an offending perpetrator. Within this exemplar, there is often a disparity between theoretical knowledge and its application in practice. Evidence relating to the non-integration of theory and practice makes the assumption, that educational dynamics may affect learning and practice outcomes and hence, the *"Gap"*. Whatever you call them, healthcare mistakes, medical errors, faults, or miscalculations. This exemplar, acknowledges that healthcare professionals and providers are provided with theoretical knowledge and prepared with skills to practice competently and safely. Yet, these same healthcare professionals and providers continue to be noncompliant with the recommended evidence-based practices which creates an ethical dilemma. Therefore, to bridge the gap between theory and practice, a *"Theory-Practice-Ethics gap"* must be considered when appraising the unacceptable outcomes in healthcare practices, and the failure of healthcare professionals and providers to fulfil their moral duty of care, as patient advocates.

One of the defining characteristics of a patient advocate is to ensure patient safety. By convention, patient advocacy is an integral philosophy in healthcare, and an obligation which is expected to be fulfilled by healthcare professionals and providers in the course of discharging their duties. *Primum non nocere 'above all, do no harm'* is a fundamental concept within the healthcare model. However, there is evidence of a failure to implement of this moral concept which relates to a patient's safety and the advocacy role expected from healthcare professionals. Healthcare professionals declare that this is because of the ambiguity associated with the comprehension of the advocacy concept in relation to the safety role. In addition to the challenge of role acceptance within a patient safety forum as a misunderstood and unappreciated responsibility. The analytical exploration of patient advocacy related to patient safety and the concept of a *"Theory-Practice-Ethics gap"* will be presented within this chapter, to reinforce the importance of their synonymous relationship for trustworthy healthcare practices. Healthcare professionals and providers need to be mindful of the importance of patient advocacy and the utilization of a safety science which leads to a higher quality of safe patient care.

Chapter 5 - Objective: Venous air embolism and hypothermia are serious and potential consequences of intravenous fluid therapy. Many patient populations may have increased risk of morbidly and mortality associated with these events. The risk management and financial impact of hospital acquired air embolism and hypothermia justifies active programs aimed at prevention. Devices used to mediate the risk of hypothermia may be sources of air embolism, making the presence of safety devices preventing infusion of air necessary.

Data Sources: The Medline publication library was used for initial literature identification.

Study Selection: A Medline publication search was conducted using keywords; air embolism, hypothermia, infusion device, inline, microbubble, transfusion cost, perioperative, prehospital, medicolegal cost.

Data Extraction and Synthesis: Publications with primary content focus of venous air embolism and hypothermia was selected for reviewed.

Conclusion: Inline fluid warming devices must employ the safest technology to ensure patients are not exposed to additional risks during active warming of infused fluids.

In: Investigating Patient Safety ISBN: 978-1-53617-344-4
Editor: Gloria Hale © 2020 Nova Science Publishers, Inc.

Chapter 1

THE ERROR AS A PARAMETER OF HEALTHCARE QUALITY

Vasiliki Kapaki[*], PhD
Faculty of Social and Political Sciences,
University of Peloponnese, Corinth, Greece

ABSTRACT

Human error is a term that is often referred to the case of an accident, whether it concerns the workplace or not. It is often used as a "causal umbrella" to easily explain an accident. The rendering of human error is preceded by the deficiencies in the system, but without necessarily incriminating the victim, since human error is considered to be a natural (albeit unpredictable) outcome of human functions, as was done previously by invoking metaphysical causes (Acts of God). So the study of human error in some cases accepted the criticism that exists to serve this purpose. Usually the "finger" shows workers and victims of accidents as the problem and therefore the most appropriate study subject as they are the ones most involved.

Indeed, the accident is the result of many interacting factors (people, materials, processes) and the attribution of causality to only one of them is an incomplete process, since taking the appropriate measures to others can

---

[*] Corresponding Author's Email: vkapaki2005@gmail.com.

be avoided. Human error cannot be independent of the system that is occurring, nor is it the only cause of an accident.

However, this does not mean that human error does not exist or is not a causal factor of accidents that should be studied. Unless the potential involuntary actions of an individual are studied, it is not possible to design the means and procedures that will prevent these actions from evolving into accidents.

The study of human error is mainly based on the science of Psychology and Mechanics and less on the Principles of Operations Research. In the chapter are summarized the main representative theories of human error such as Bad Apples Theory, Normal Accident Theories and High Reliability Organizations Theory etc.

Keywords: bad apples theory, normal accident theories, high reliability organizations theory, 1st and 2nd generation human error models

ABBREVIATIONS

ATHEANA	A Technique for Human Error Analysis
CREAM	Cognitive Reliability and Error Analysis Method
HCR	Human Cognitive Reliability (Model)
HEART	Human Error Assessment and Reduction Technique;
HERMES	Human Error Risk Management for Engineering Systems (Model)
HF/E	Human Factors/Ergonomics (Model)
HROT	High Reliability Organizations Theory
IDAC	Information – Decision – Action - Crew (Model)
IOM	Institution of Medicine
SHARP	Systematic Human Action Reliability Procedure
SLIM	Success Likelihood Index Method
SRK	Skill Rule Knowledge (Model)
TALENT	Task Analysis – Linked Evaluation Technique
THERP	Technique Human Error Rate Prediction (Model)
TRC	Time Reliability Correlation (Model)

INTRODUCTION

Human factors are an established scientific discipline used in a large number of other safety crucial industries. Human factors approaches underpin at present patient safety and quality improvement science, offering an integrated, evidenced and coherent approach to patient safety, quality improvement and clinical excellence.

The practices of human factors focus on making optimal human performance through better understanding the individuals' behavior, their interactions with each other and with their environment. By acknowledging human limitations, human factors offers ways to trivialize and become less severe human frailties, so reducing adverse events and medical errors and its consequences. The system-wide adoption of these concepts offers a without parallel opportunity to support cultural change and empower the healthcare systems to put patient safety and clinical excellence at their heart. Human factors principles can be applied in the identification, assessment and management of patient safety risks, and in the analysis of incidents to identify learning and corrective actions.

In general, human factors knowledge and techniques can be used to notify quality betterment in teams and services, support change management, and help to say more loudly the importance of the design of equipment and procedures (Carayon et al., 2014).

CONCEPTUAL CLARIFICATION OF TERMS "ERROR" AND "MISTAKE"

It is difficult to give a precise definition of the human error especially when such a definition is intended for scientific study. In fact, this concept has three different aspects (Hollnagel, 2005):

- Cause: error in this case is an action or omission that caused an adverse effect, namely it is the cause.

- Fact or action: in this case the interest is focused on the action or the omission itself without taking under consideration the effect.
- Consequence: in this case interest is solely focused on the effect which is repeated with the action.

In general, human error that leads to an adverse effect is not easily and always observable, because it is not always an intentional action or a consequence thereof (Hollnagel, 1983). The attribution of liability for the error to an individual or a group constitutes a psychosocial process which may easily become vulnerable to opinions, attitudes and interests and not an objective technical process. This subjective process usually aims at finding an "acceptable cause" which must have the following characteristics (Hollnagel, 2005):

- To be inarguably associated with the system's structure or operation, so that the cause will be directly associated with the system itself and to be able to be corrected with actions completed internally by it. The attribution of liability to external and uncontrolled factors is not satisfactory, because if the system cannot protect itself by such uncontrollable mechanisms, it means that the level of prevention measures is not high.
- To be manageable given the resources and the time, so as not to exceed internal capabilities for its correction. The attribution of liability for problems that require excessive resources or time is not satisfactory, since better protection measures should be involved.
- To comply with the existing rules of justification, namely with the acceptable theory regarding the system's rules and operation. In the event that the justification conflicts with the system's rules and philosophy or it can not be interpreted according to them, the explanation is not accepted.

Reason defines error as a general term in order to include all those cases in which a scheduled process of mental or physical activities fails to achieve the desired result and this failure cannot be attributed to random facts. He mentions three types of errors (Reason, 2000):

- The slips, which are errors in the execution of an appropriate plan or unintended actions.
- The lapses are errors that refer to an intended action that was not performed due to memory failure.
- The mistakes, which are errors manifested in the design of the action plan.

In its report on medical errors published in 2000, the Institute of Medicine (IOM) defines as an error the unsuccessful completion of a planned action or the implementation of an incorrect planning for the achievement of a goal (Institute of Medicine Committee on Quality of Health Care in, 2000).

According to Leape, the term error refers to an unnecessary action which takes place or it is omitted or an action which eventually did not bring the desired result (Leape, 1994). Respectively, other authors, refer to error as an unsuccessful action regardless of the imminent damages (Hofer, Kerr, and Hayward, 2000).

At the same time, international literature does not provide a commonly accepted definition for the word error, which justifies the interchangeable use of the terms error and mistake for similar issues without a clear distinction between the two concepts.

The difficulty to provide a precise conceptual clarification of the term "error" as well as the subjective aspect thereof results to the development of different and conflicting theories and models or methods designed to manage human errors especially in high-risk areas. In the following sections of this chapter there it is attempted to present the models developed for the management of human errors.

THE ROLE OF HUMAN ERRORS IN ELICITING ADVERSE EVENTS

The subjectivity of human errors gives rise to the presentation of different opinions regarding its involvement in eliciting adverse events. According to the scientific literature, it is claimed that 90% (Technica, 1989) or 66% (Williamson and Feyer, 1990) or a percentage between 50% and 80% (Hollnagel, 1998 andRasmussen, 1983) of the accidents include error data attributed to human factors. The main reasons for this increased percentage are (Cacciabue, 1998):

- The reliability of the technological equipment which is enhanced due to the technological development.
- The multilevel and complex nature of the system and man's involvement in it.

However, there are opposing views according to which it is estimated that 80% of the accidents in complex systems is linked to system problems and 20% is caused by human actions (Livingston, Jackson, and Priestley, 2001). Similar is the opinion of Bellamy and Geyer, according to who, the involvement of human factor in accidents amounts to 25% (Bellamy and Geyer, 1992). Over the last few years there has been a serious progress in the development of security systems that already take precautionary measures in order to address human errors, specified as a probability and therefore not a cause of failure.

Rassmussen, argues that it is difficult to estimate the involvement of human error in adverse events since (Rasmussen, 1983):

- Adverse events and accidents which are demonstrably attributed to human errors are very few but must be examined due to the importance of their consequences. Low probability for an accident attributed to a human error does not allow for an appropriate statistical study and precise conclusions, due to lack of adequate facts.

- Systems' complexity contributed to the increase of the required time and facts in order to examine a system, but they also change very rapidly therefore reducing the available time for their study.

In conclusion, the subjectivity of the process that causes human errors does not facilitate the attribution of a precise human error causality rate to adverse events. The role of human errors in eliciting accidents is a fact but there is also human involvement.

THEORETICAL APPROACHES TO HUMAN ERROR

The study of human error is mainly based on the science of Psychology and Mechanics and less on the principles of operational investigation. A summary of three representative theories on human errors is presented below.

Bad Apples Theory

According to this theory, if an employee makes a mistake in the course of their work, they are automatically characterized as insufficient and must be immediately removed from the working field so as not to impede the proper function of the organization or influence negatively the work of the rest of the employees. This theory is based on three assumptions (Shojania and Dixon-Woods, 2013):

- Complex systems usually fail due to people's unpredictable behavior.
- Human errors cause accidents.
- Failures are unexpected.

Berwick argues that this theory is based on Quality Assurance. However, this fact cannot be proved, since if this were true, the dismissal of workers who commit errors would automatically mean complete elimination of errors and adverse events. But this is not the case (Berwick, 1989).

Normal Accident Theory

According to this theory, errors and accidents constitute a fundamental characteristic of complex systems. In accordance with Perrow the more complex a system is, the more likely it is to cause an adverse event. In order to describe adverse events, Perrow introduced the concept of "accident," urged by the accident that took place in 1979 in USA at the Nuclear Energy Station "Three Mile Island" (Perrow, 1984). This theory is also supported by Reason, who argues that the more complex a system is, it is more likely to lead to adverse events. His theory explains the multiple and highly reliable methods for detecting, reporting and listing an error in complex systems (Reason, 1990).

High Reliability Organizations Theory (HROT)

The concept of security policy becomes more interesting in High Risk Organizations, and High Reliability Organizations. According to this theory organizational structure as well as the corporate culture of these organizations is based on security and aim at reducing the probability of an error. In these organizations (i.e., airline companies, nuclear stations etc.) the safety of products or services provided is a priority due to the disastrous consequences of a possible error. For example, the collision of Air France Concorde aircraft in 2000 near the airport Charles de Gaulle due to a fire in the engine, resulted to the death of 110 passengers and the disruption of aircraft traffic of the said company around the world, under the weight of public opinion reactions (La Porte and Rochlin, 1994, Roberts 1990, Roberts, Stout, and Halpern, 1994, Rochlin, LaPorte, and Roberts, 1987).

1ST AND 2ND GENERATION HUMAN ERROR MODELS

Most of the researchers divide human errors into two main groups (Lees, 1996):

- Errors associated with human behavior.
- Errors associated with the context within the error occur.

Cacciabue has a similar opinion, that there are two categories of errors (Cacciabue, 1992):

- The errors related to the human factor (behavioral approach). This approach is based on the model of Behavioral Psychology according to which the human brain is compared to a "black box" in which stimuli are inserted and reactions are educed/evoked regardless of the context, therefore it is likely for an error to be predicted based on a statistic analysis, provided that several behavioral studies have been made in advance.
- Errors associated with the system itself and the working conditions.

According to the two aforementioned approaches of the human error there are models based more on the one or the other approach consisting of elements from both approaches.

Behavioral models approach human error as an issue of human behavior and try to improve it by modifying it (Cacciabue, 1998 andLees, 1996). According to these models, errors are categorized into errors of omission that refer to the non-execution of the indicated action, errors of commission which are associated with wrong choices – actions that impede the situation and irrelevant actions (Apostolakis 2004 and Dougherty, 1993).

Time models address human error as a time variable that results from natural variability of human behavior therefore following a distribution curve in relation to time. It is an inevitable phenomenon therefore emphasis is placed on the possibility of remedying (despite its prevention), which also depends on the available time (Swain, 1990).

The Human Factors/Ergonomics – HF/E Models are based on human-machine interaction and approach human error as a result of the working conditions that they try to improve. In general, frame models examine the relationship between the type of the error and the characteristics of work. A disadvantage of these models is the failure to explain how same or similar situations lead to different forms of error (Reason, 1990).

The models of cognitive mechanics are simple and clearly present the framework, taking under consideration the working conditions but they focus on the cognitive factors. They emphasize on the relationship between the type of errors and the causes thereof (Lees, 1996).

Along with the aforementioned models, various techniques have been developed for the quantification of human error, which can be grouped into three categories:

- *Synthetic or Analytic methods:* They are based on the analysis of tasks into elementary tasks and collection of historical data regarding the human behavior failure rate in them. This way the probability of failure in elementary tasks is estimated. The probability of more complex tasks is then estimated with a linear combination of the elementary tasks in a sequence. The analysis of tasks into elements and the attribution of error probabilities to every element has been criticized on the grounds that it doesn't take under consideration an internal mental model or cognitive processes and therefore it is not easy to explain why similar situations lead to different outcomes (Hollnagel, 1992b). These methods also don't take under consideration influencing factors such as noise, which may sometimes elicit the cause or become the cause. A simple individual error can hardly lead to accidents by itself due to the existence of safety factors (Hollnagel, 1998). Human errors are not independent individual facts but they are interlinked with the situations they create and other events in the system (Bersini, Cacciabue and Mancini, 1988). Therefore, the error is a set of many circumstances.

- *Typical Reliability Methods:* Error in this category of methods is considered as a phenomenon that mainly depends on time or the number of times that a process is repeated. On the contrary to machine failures people can correct their errors and this fact must be taken under consideration in the evaluation of human reliability (Hollnagel, 1998).
- *Subjective Specialists Judgments:* These are made immediately by specialists for the whole process followed by an appropriate statistical processing. The probability is directly evaluated by specialists and immediate conclusions are drawn (Hollnagel, 1998).

These techniques have been heavily criticized. However, it is worth noting that regardless of the technical method used, all of them involve the subjective judgement of the analyst.

1st Generation Models of Human Error - Behavioral Models

The characteristic of these models is analysis into elementary stimulus-reaction pairs followed by the algebraic combination thereof in order to be elevated to integrated operations or tasks. Therefore, the systematic observations of users have led to the following conclusions (Tanaka et al., 1989):

- Individuals tend switch to the final stage of the task, overlooking the intermediate stages that present less interest in relation to the result.
- Individuals tend to postpone actions that they deem as not very important.
- The more important the action is considered by the individuals the less are the derogations observed throughout the daily process.

Technique for Human Error Rate Prediction (THERP) MODEL
This model was developed in the USA between 1970 and 1980, implementing a digital logic, it is an analytic-synthetic model. It starts with

an activity analysis, breaking them down to elementary activities and then describing them through event-trees. Then follows an algebraic synthesis of error probabilities per activity as conditional probabilities from the partial probabilities of the elementary operations (Lees, 1996).

Times Models

In time models error usually results from the variability of performance, which sometimes lies outside the bounds and is enough to lead the whole system to failure (Hudoklin and Rozman, 1992 andSwain, 1990). Small off-limits derogations, are not only inevitable, but also desired since small off-limits derogations are necessary in order to expand the boundaries. Therefore, if this variability leads to positive outcomes, it is characterized as creativity and learning whereas, if the outcomes are negative, it is characterized as human error (Hollnagel, 2002). The approach of a difficult situation initially starts with error detections, followed by error diagnosis and then the correction thereof.

Time – Reliability Correlation (TRC) Model

According to this model, although there are many factors that influence performance, time is the most important of them. It expresses the probability of failure as a function of time. The underlying assumption behind Time-Reliability Correlation was that the longer the available time for diagnosis is the greater is the reliability (Fujita, 1992). This model draws on the conclusions from the education with the use of simulators in order to create a group of time-reliability correlation curves. Then these curves are adjusted using Scalable Link Interface, SLI and other specialist approaches to particular circumstances (Fragola and Dougherty, 1988).

The main disadvantage of this model is the failure to explain the reasons behind a particular behavior and what triggered it.

Error Correction Model

This model focuses on error correction whenever this is possible. According to this model an error is not dangerous if the system gives the individual the opportunity to correct it in time. Correction mechanisms include (Moray and Dougherty, 1990):

- Human actions if the activity is controlled by another individual.
- States of the system (indications).
- States of the equipment (active – targeted and passive – general inspections)

It is economically expedient to adopt error correction strategies rather than expensive precaution measures.

Frame – Ergonomic Models

A typical feature of these models is that human error cannot be predicted and it is the result of the men interaction with the immediate environment. The possibility of error according to this model emerges only if the ability of the user is downgraded either due to a mental factor or because of an undesired external condition. Just like behavioral models, ergonomic models implement an analytical property, namely the ability to analyze the system in additional unique elements, whose error probabilities, when aggregated, equal the overall error probability of the system (Cacciabue, 1992).

Success Likelihood Index Method (SLIM)

This method examines not only the quality of the factors that influence the performance but also the importance of their effect. The basic principle of this method is that a possible error in a particular situation depends on the combined effect of relevant few factors that influence performance either human or associated with the working conditions (Lees, 1996).

Human Error Assessment and Reduction Technique (HEART)

The probability of error in this technique is approached as a function of the type of the activity and the relevant influencing factors. Human reliability is considered directly dependent on performance influencing factors (Jo and Park, 2003).

Cognitive Models

According to these models, the difficulty to predict human error results from the lack of knowledge and not the existence of randomness. According to the supporters of cognitive approaches the causes of errors are the following (Bersini, Cacciabue, and Mancini, 1988 and Hollnagel, 1992b):

- Incompatibility between the user's knowledge and the required knowledge (abilities). Various levels of specialization among various people also lead to different approaches to the solution of problems. A particular task may be simple for a person but complex for a less skilled person. The definition of a simple or complex task depends on the person and the situation.
- Inaccurate execution of plans which may be caused either by the difference between the actual conditions and the model of representation that an individual has for itself (systemic errors), or by random variations as a result of brain function, small influences from the environment, loss of memory or attention etc. which refer to errors of omission or practical errors.

Skill - Rule – Knowledge (SRK) Model

Rasmussen's Skill – Rule – Knowledge model, is the most debated model in the literature regarding the approach of human error. According to Rasmussen, there are three types of human behavior (Rasmussen, 1983):

- Skill – based behavior that occurs without deliberate attention and it is based on facts.
- Rule – based behavior that is deliberately controlled and it is focused on specific objectives.
- Knowledge – based behavior that is also deliberately controlled but also involves justification.

Apart from the behavior this model also emphasizes on the information, therefore distinguishing between three types of information (Hale, 1990):

- A signal is simply perceived as a continuous quantitative indicator of the state of the system.
- A sign is perceived as an indication of a distinct state and many times as the need to take action.
- A symbol is related to the system's functional property.

The main source of errors is associated with modifications in working environment that requires changes in the behavior of the employees. Every alteration to the system such as the introduction of a new technology inevitably alters working conditions for the people involved in the system and therefore their mental functions. A crucial factor for the elimination of errors is the one that ensures an appropriate level of operation at the appropriate time (Hale, 1990).

Human Cognitive Reliability (HCR) Model
This model constitutes a combination of SRK and the ability to quantify TRC. The purpose of this model is to politicize the probabilities of human error regardless of time. It has been heavily criticized mainly in relation to two points (Fujita, 1992):

- It doesn't have a stable psychological basis therefore it is impossible to differentiate in separate cognitive processes that lead to the same time of response and it cannot tackle sudden changes on the level of behavior based on skill, rules and knowledge.
- It cannot examine practical errors that occur throughout the diagnosis and phenomena, where error probability increases over completion time. Practical errors can be predicted to a certain point but that doesn't apply to the omissions, since lack of attention is likely to occur at any time.

Absentmindeism Model
Reason's absentmindeism model, is one of the most popular models along with Rasmussen's SRK model. In this model Reason categorizes errors in slips, lapses and mistakes. The term slip, refers to an error

committed throughout the implementation of an appropriate plan, or to an involuntary action. The term laps, refers to an error where a deliberate action was not performed due to memory failure and finally the term mistake refers to an error in the determination of an action plan i.e., diagnosis, planning etc. Reason, also refers to the concept of "violation" which is a deliberate action that pursues the appropriate purposes but defies a standard, process or practice. Violations are not examined in literature due to the peculiarities they present.

Respectively to error categories the model also determines the main categories of "internal error standards" during planning, saving and execution which are respectively associated with faults, omissions, and slips. Slips and omissions may be corrected relatively easier than faults since they are detected in the stages of execution and completion, whereas errors are detected in the stage of completion whenever an undesirable outcome is observed.

Based on Rasmussen's model, Reason attempted to associate omissions, slips and faults with the levels of behavior referred to in Rasmussen's model (Rasmussen, 1982 andReason, 1990).

Human Error Risk Management for Engineering Systems (HERMES) Model

This model attempts to take under consideration the points of view and determine a chronological and logical sequence for evaluation of danger. HERMES method aims to understand the mechanisms (Cacciabue, 2004).

Task Analysis – Linked Evaluation Technique (TALENT)

This model is based on the assumption that in complex systems and particularly in very stressful period's individuals is led to action or inactivity mainly due to latent and cognitive or behavioral and social factors rather than factors relevant to the equipment. According to this model individuals behave like human beings with a free will (Ryan, 1988, 1990).

Systematic Human Action Reliability Procedure (SHARP)

This method adopts simultaneously both HCR and THERP methods for the evaluation of cognitive and procedural errors respectively. It acknowledges two levels of user behavior (Bersini, Cacciabue, and Mancini, 1988):

- The first high level of decision making allows for the utilization of user's knowledge who constantly identifies situations and develops audit and supervisory strategies. It is clearly a cognitive function without immediate interaction with the actual control system. Diagnosis and planning operate in parallel.
- The second low level of decision making is supported by the potential working and conscious memory, when the user implements a prescheduled response or a planned strategy in order to meet a specific objective.

At the level of decision making the planning process is based on three knowledge bases (Bersini, Cacciabue, and Mancini, 1988):

- On the basis of objective knowledge (it includes all the goals that the user may achieve).
- On the basis of system knowledge (which includes the structural representation of the system).
- On the basis of process knowledge (which includes the data used to assimilate the representation of natural phenomena in user's mind).

The low level of decision-making focuses on the interaction between the user and the system (Bersini, Cacciabue, and Mancini, 1988).

Supply – Demand Imbalance Model

The supply-demand imbalance model examines human error as a result of imbalance between the requirements of the task and the performer's skills (Lees, 1996). Every task requires certain skills and competences that individuals possess to a different extent. The difference between the required level or working skills and the available level of the user's working skills determines the probability of an error. Therefore, the complexity of the task plays a key role. The subjective and objective features of a complex task have raised serious concerns in literature. According to Campbell, the subjective features are the following (Campbell, 1988):

- The psychological experience of the individual that performs the task.
- The interaction between the task and the characteristics of the individual that performs the task. The tasks are more or less complex depending on the abilities of the individuals who perform the tasks.
- A result of the objective characteristics of the task. More specifically, complex tasks are characterized by unknown or uncertain consequences. The relationship between the medium and the objective is unknown in complex tasks. Finally, complex tasks may be divided into additional individual sections.

Apart from the subjective features of a complex task, Campbell also acknowledges the objective features of complex tasks such as (Campbell, 1988):

- Multiple probable ways to achieve the desirable outcome therefore multiple information.
- Multiple results.
- Opposite interactions between routes.
- Correlation between probable existing characteristics of the task, such as the lack of structure in the objective complexity of a task.

This model fails to explain why individuals may sometimes perform an error and not every time. Additionally, it is hard to define and measure the skills of an individual since they constitute qualitative characteristics.

Approaches to Information Processing

According to these models, human error refers to the way information is being received and transmitted as well as processed. It is therefore a brain overload problem or a problem of communication between the transmitter (sender) and the receiver (audience). According to communication management models, the type of error generally depends on information management (Hollnagel, 1992a). More specifically:

- If the priority is to complete an activity without being interrupted by other events, the outcome shall be an error of omission.
- If the priority is to reduce the completion time of the current activity, the error is associated with the decrease of accuracy.
- If the priority is not to lose any information, in this case the error refers to the creation of anticipation.

Transmitter – receiver communication constitutes another category of error that is analyzed by Communication process models (Bellamy, 1983).

Socio-Technical Systems

The models of these systems highlight the key role of organizational and broader socio-technical factors in human error. Complex systems consist of groups of individuals which play a dominant role in systems security. Team attitude is influenced not only by the cognitive processes of each individual but also by the communication and cooperation between them (Lees, 1996). In the models of this category there are two significant concepts that play a key role. These are the concepts of team thinking and the concept of dependence.

Team thinking is the phenomenon whereby people share the judgment of another individual without too much thought. A similar phenomenon occurs when an individual that has made a mistake repeats it, because it has been persuaded that it must be the correct "mind set." Error in these cases cannot be corrected because it is shared by others without thinking (Greenstreet Berman Ltd, 2001).

The dependence of human error is associated with the state, in which some sort of personal or external factor establishes a relationship between two independent actions. There are two types of dependence (Greenstreet Berman Ltd, 2001):

- Errors of common cause, in which case employees perform the same error or different errors due to poor education or poorly designed systems.
- Human errors caused by dependence, in which case human action creates a dependency between two or more independent systems, such as a not well-trained technician who performs the same error in all parallel systems.

2nd Generation Models of Human Error

Information – Decision – Action – Crew (IDAC) Model

This is a causal model, according to which error makes sense only within the framework in which it occurs. IDAC model consists of additional models of information processing (Information), problem solving and decision making (Decision) and Action of the Crew, after whom it has been named (Mosleh and Chang, 2004).

- Model "I" refers to information perception, comparison, removal and grouping and consists of three types of memory: Work memory, Intermediate Memory, "Knowledge-based" Memory
- Model "D" includes not only decision-making strategies but also decision making and matches diagnosis and activity planning.

Model IDAC takes under consideration both mental states, namely the individual's feelings towards a stimulus as well as the personal characteristics and the impact of the group.

Cognitive Reliability and Error Analysis Method (CREAM)

This method presents an error classification system that includes individual, technological, and organizational factors. According to it human performance depends largely on the situation and distinguishes among four levels of individual's control on the task performed (Hollnagel, 1992a, Hollnagel, 1998 andKonstantinidou et al., 2006):

- At irregular control level the selection of the next action is random. There is no significant relation between the situation and the actions. This is usually the case when individuals are panicked.
- At occasional control level, next action is defined by obvious characteristics. It is performed due to inadequate level of information regarding a situation or due to lack of skills and knowledge or due to unusual environment conditions. The selection in this case is usually ineffective (error).
- At regular control level, performance follows a more or less familiar process or rule.
- At strategic level, performance is planned for a longer term with strategic objectives. Multiple and higher-level objectives and operational interactions are usually included.

A Technique for Human Error Analysis (ATHEANA)

This method examines people-centered factors as well as the system conditions that cause the need for action and interaction. ATHEANA method is based on judgments regarding the evaluation of error probability for a specific framework and activity.

Accidents constitute a complex phenomenon which is based on both men and their environment. Their main component is the risk that involves the mechanisms of what is inherently unknown, which have to be confronted by individuals in every action they take, every minute of their lives (Konstantinidou et al., 2006).

CONCLUSION

Innate ignorance is, however, not capable to prevent human creativity. Knowledge has always been a virtue that men gradually had to build up by using imperfect models that succeeded each other. Therefore, up to date it never acquired complete knowledge of a mechanism, but only better approaches and mental constructions that help individuals to better manage ignorance regarding the universe, while reaching closer to the truth.

In the case of accidents, the concept of flawlessly repeated situations is far from the truth, since it is a rare phenomenon that is not often repeated and surely not under the same conditions. It is probably limited to its intuitive nature and therefore better matches the concept of uncertainty, since it is ignorance of the mechanisms and not ignorance of the outcomes with a certain analogy.

REFERENCES

Apostolakis, G. E. (2004). "How useful is Quantitative Risk assessment? ." *Risk Analysis* no. 24 (3):515-520.

Bellamy, L. J. (1983). "Neglected Individual, Social and Organisational Factors." *Reliability Engineering and System Safety* no. 83:2B/5/1.

Bellamy, L. J.and Geyer, T. A. W. (1992). Organisational, Management and Human Factor in Quantified Risk Assessment. . In *HSE Contract Research Report*. UK.

Bersini, U., Cacciabue, P. C. and Mancini, G. (1988). "Cognitive Modelling: A basic complement of Human Reliability Analysis." *Reliability Engineering and System Safety* no. 22:107-128.

Berwick, D. M. (1989). "Continuous improvement as an ideal in health care." *N Engl J Med* no. 320 (1):53-6. doi: 10.1056/nejm 198901053200110.

Cacciabue, P. C. (1992). "Cognitive Modelling: A fundamental issue for Human Reliability Assessment Methodology?" *Reliability Engineering and System safety* no. 38:91-97.

Cacciabue, P. C. (1998). "Modelling and simulation of human behaviour for safety analysis and control of complex systems." *Safety Science* no. 28 (2):97-110. doi: http://dx.doi.org/10.1016/S0925-7535(97)00079-9.

Cacciabue, P. C. (2004). "Human Error Risk Management for Engineering Systems: A methodology for design, safety assessment, accident investigation and training." *Reliability Engineering and System Safety* no. 83:229-240.

Campbell, D. J. (1988). "Task Complexity: A review and analysis." *Academy of Management Review* no. 13 (1):40-52.

Carayon, P., Tosha, B. W., Rivera-Rodriguez, A. J., Schoofs Hundt, A., Hoonakker,, P., Holden R.and Gurses, A. P. (2014). "Human factors systems approach to healthcare quality and patient safety." *Applied ergonomics* no. 45 (1):14-25. doi: 10.1016/j.apergo.2013.04.023.

Dougherty, E. M. (1993). "Context and Human Reliability Analysis." *Reliability Engineering and System safety* no. 41:25-47.

Fragola, J. R. and Dougherty, E. M. (1988). "Human Reliability Analysis." *Jouhn-Wiley Inter Science*.

Fujita, Y. (1992). "Human Reliability Analysis: A human point of view." *Reliability Engineering and System Safety* no. 38:71-79.

Greenstreet Berman Ltd. (2001). Preventing the propagation of error and misplaced reliance on faulty systems: A guide to human error dependency. In *Offshore Technology Report 2001/053*.

Hale, A. R. (1990). "How people learn to live with risk: Prediction and Control." *Journal of Occupational Accidents* no. 13:33-45.

Hofer, T. P., Kerr, E. A. and Hayward, R. A. (2000). "What is an error?" *Eff Clin Pract* no. 3 (6):261-9.

Hollnagel, E. (1992a). *Coping, Coupling and Control: The Modelling of Muddling Through*. Paper read at 2nd Interdisciplinary Workshop on Mental Models, at Cambridge, UK.

Hollnagel, E. (1992b). "The Reliability of Man - Machine Interaction." *Reliability Engineering and System safety* no. 38:81-89.

Hollnagel, E. (2002). Barrier Analysis and Accident Prevention. In *2002 Human Technology Integration Colloquium Series*: Air Force Research Laboratory, Human Effectiveness Directorate.

Hollnagel, E. (2005). *The Elusiveness of "Human Error"* [cited 14.06.2014. Available from http://www.humanerroranalysis.com/page/on-human-error-the-elusiveness-of-human-error.

Hollnagel, E. (1983). *Position paper on human error. Responses to Queries from the Program Committee.* Paper read at NATO Conference on Human Error, September 5-9,, at Bellagio, Italy,.

Hollnagel, E. (1998). "Chapter 1 - The State of Human Reliability Analysis." In *Cognitive Reliability and Error Analysis Method (CREAM)*, edited by Erik Hollnagel, 1-21. Oxford: Elsevier Science Ltd.

Hudoklin, A. and Rozman, V. (1992). "Human Errors versus Stress." *Reliability Engineering and System Safety* no. 37:231-236.

Institute of Medicine Committee on Quality of Health Care in, America. 2000. *To Err is Human: Building a Safer Health System*, edited by L. T. Kohn, J. M. Corrigan and M. S. Donaldson. Washington (DC): National Academies Press (US) Copyright 2000 by the National Academy of Sciences. All rights reserved.

Jo, Y. D. and Park, K. S. (2003). "Dynamic management of human error to reduce total risks." *Journal of Loss Prevention on the Process Industries* no. 16:313-321.

Konstantinidou, M., Nivolianitou, Z., Kiranoudis, C. and Markatos, N. (2006). "A fuzzy modeling application of CREAM methodology for human reliability analysis." *Reliability Engineering and System Safety* no. 91:706-716.

La Porte, T. R.and Rochlin, G. I. (1994). "A rejoinder to Perrow." *J Conting Crisis Manage* no. 2:221-227.

Leape, L. L. (1994). "Error in medicine." *Jama* no. 272 (23):1851-7.

Lees, P. F. (1996). *Loss prevention in the process industries.* 2nd ed: Reed Educational and Professional Publishing.

Livingston, A. D., Jackson, G. and Priestley, K. (2001). Root Causes Analysis: Literature Review. In *HSE Contract Research Report. 325/2001.* UK.

Moray, N. and Dougherty, E. M. (1990). "Dilemma and the One-sidedness of Human Reliability Analysis." *Reliability Engineering and System Safety* no. 29:337-344.

Mosleh, A.and Chang, Y. (2004). "Model -based human reliability analysis: prospects and requirements." *Reliability Engineering and System Safety* no. 83:241-253.

Perrow, C. (1984). *Normal Accidents*. Edited by Living with High-Risk Technologies. New York: Basic Books. Reprint, 2nd.

Rasmussen, J. (1982). "Human Errors. A taxonomy for describing human malfunction in Industrial Installations." *Journal of Occupational Accidents*. no. 4:331-333.

Rasmussen, J. (1983). Skills, Rules, Knowledge: Signals, Signs and Symbols and other distinctions in Human Performance Models. In *IEEE Trans. Syst. Man Cybern*.

Reason, J. (1990). *Human Error*: Cambridge University Press.

Reason, J. (2000). "Human error: models and management." *Bmj* no. 320 (7237):768-70.

Roberts, K. H. (1990). "Some characteristics of high reliability organizations." *Org. Sci* no. 1:160-177.

Roberts, K. H., Stout, S. K. and Halpern, J. J. (1994). "Decision dynamics in two high reliability military organizations" *Manage Sci* no. 40:614-624.

Rochlin, G. I., LaPorte, T. R. and Roberts, K. H. (1987). "The self-designing high reliability organization. Aircraft carrier flight operations at sea." *Naval War College Review* no. 42:76-90.

Ryan, T. G. (1988). "Task Analysis - Linked Approach for Integrating the Human Factors in Reliability Assessments of Nuclear Power Plants (TALENT)." *Reliability Engineering and System safety* no. 22:219-234.

Ryan, T. G. (1990). "Human Reliability Analysis - Why not turn to the human factors community?" *Reliability Engineering and System Safety* no. 29:345-358.

Shojania, K. G. and Dixon-Woods, M. (2013). "'Bad apples': time to redefine as a type of systems problem?" *BMJ Qual Saf* no. 22 (7):528-31. doi: 10.1136/bmjqs-2013-002138.

Swain, A. D. (1990). "Human reliability analysis: Need, Status, Trends and Limitations." *Reliability Engineering and System Safety* no. 29:301-313.

Tanaka, I., Kimura, T., Utsunomiya, S., Uno, K., Endo, T., Tani, M., Fujita, Y., Kurimoto, A., Mikami, A., Kishimoto, N., Narikuni, K., Kawamura, M.,Kubo, S., Maeyama, K., Ishigaki, N., Tsukumoto, T., Nishimura, Y., Morita, A., Shono, M. and Morita, M. (1989). *Studies of Operator*

Human Reliability Using Training Simulator (1)-(5). Paper read at 1989 Fall Meeting on the Atomic Energy Society of Japan, at Tokai, Japan,.

Technica. (1989). *Evaluation of the Human Contribution to Pipework and In - Line Equipment Failure Frequencies*. London: UK Health and Safety Executive.

Williamson, A. and Feyer, A. M. (1990). "Behavioural Epidemiology as a Tool for Accident Research" *Journal of Occupational Accidents* no. 12:207-222.

BIOGRAPHICAL SKETCH

Vasiliki Kapaki

Affiliation:
Faculty of Social and Political Sciences, University of Peloponnese, Corinth, Greece Education:

- Postdoctoral Research Fellow in Health Economics, University of Peloponnese, Corinth Greece
- Doctor of Philosophy – PhD in Health Policy - Quality of HealthCare Services and Patient Safety, University of Peloponnese, Corinth Greece
- Master of Science (MSc) in Health Economics and Management, University of Piraeus, Greece
- Bachelor in Social Policy, Panteion University, Athens, Greece

Business Address:
44-46 Kriton street, 117 44, Athens, Greece

Research and Professional Experience:

- Consulting Services in Health Policy, Health Economics, Pharmacoeconomics, Health Technology Assessment (HTA) and Real World Evidence (RWE)

- Quality of Healthcare Services
- Total Quality Management
- Patient Safety
- Drug Safety
- Risk Management in Healthcare Organizations (adverse events, medical errors and near misses management)

Professional Appointments:

- Nov. 2018- Jan. 2020 : Scientific Member of the Greek Health Technology Assessment Committee (G-HTA)
- 2016- present: Postdoctoral Research Fellow in Health Economics, University of Peloponnese, Corinth, Greece
- 2015-Sep.2018: External Health Policy Consultant, Institute of Health Policy, Athens, Greece
- 2015-present: Teaching and Research Staff in Postgraduate programs in University of Peloponnese, Corinth, Greece and in Medical School of National and Kapodistrian University of Athens, Greece
- 2014-2015: Research Fellow in Health Policy, University of Peloponnese, Corinth, Greece
- 2010-2013: Research Fellow in Health Policy and Health Economics, National School of Public Health, Athens, Greece
- Souliotis K, Golna C, Kotsopoulos N, Kapaki V, Dalucas C. (2018). Meningitis B vaccination: knowledge and attitudes of pediatricians and parents in Greece. Heliyon;11;4(11):e00902.
- Kapaki, V. (2018). The anatomy of medication errors. In Dr. Stanislaw Stawicki (Ed.), Vignettes in Patient Safety - Volume 4. ISBN 978-953-51-6916-1.
- Kapaki, V. & Souliotis, K. (2018). Defining adverse events and determinants of medical errors in healthcare. In Dr. Stanislaw Stawicki (Ed.), Vignettes in Patient Safety - Volume 3. ISBN 978-953-51-6155-4.

- Kapaki, V. & Souliotis, K. (2017). Psychometric properties of the Hospital Survey on Patient Safety Culture (HSOPSC): Findings from Greece. In M. S. Firstenberg and S. P. Stawicki (Ed.), Vignettes in Patient Safety - Volume 2. ISBN 978-953-51-5757-1.
- Kapaki, V. & Souliotis, K. (2017). Patient Safety and Medical Errors: Building Safer Healthcare Systems for Better Care. In M. Riga (Ed.), Impact of Medical Errors and Malpractice on Health Economics, Quality, and Patient Safety (pp. 61-90). Hershey, PA: IGI Global.doi:10.4018/978-1-5225-2337-6.ch003.
- Kapaki, V. & Souliotis, K. (2017). Patient Safety Culture in Greece: Narrowing the Gap between the Principles of Patient Safety Culture and Current Clinical Practice. In E.Williams (Ed.), Patient Safety and Management: Perspectives, Principles and Emerging Issues (pp. 87-117). Nova Science Publisher Inc.

In: Investigating Patient Safety
Editor: Gloria Hale
ISBN: 978-1-53617-344-4
© 2020 Nova Science Publishers, Inc.

Chapter 2

PURSUING PATIENT SAFETY THROUGH RESEARCHING AND REDUCING DIAGNOSTIC ERRORS AND APPLYING A SYSTEMATIC APPROACH TO DIAGNOSIS

Ami Schattner[*], *MD*
The Faculty of Medicine, Hebrew University and Hadassah Medical School, Jerusalem, Israel

ABSTRACT

Adverse patient outcomes, including mortality, are often associated with iatrogenic harm. While medication errors, health care-associated infections and falls have long been the focus of attention and a well-established target of intervention, diagnostic errors have been relatively neglected. Nevertheless, errors in diagnosis (including incorrect, missed or

---

[*] Corresponding Author's Email: amischatt@gmail.com.

delayed diagnosis) constitute an important facet of patient safety, and may also be preventable.

In contrast with the prevailing view that advances in scientific knowledge and technology have practically eliminated the possibility of errors in diagnosis, data from autopsy studies, readmissions research and claims data reveal that these errors continue to occur with an estimated incidence of 10-20% and not infrequently, dire consequences. Therefore, further study is required to illuminate the multifactorial origins of diagnostic errors and develop techniques for improving clinical reasoning and the diagnostic process thereby reducing unwanted errors.

We define mistakes in the diagnostic process, identify their major causes, and suggest several principles of optimal, bias-free diagnosis based on the SOAP mnemonic stressing a Systematic methodical approach, Observation and listening to the patient, Accessing databases for patient-tailored decisions, and adopting a Personal, humanistic, patient-centered communication to reduce diagnostic errors and enhance patient safety.

INTRODUCTION

Improving patient safety mandates identification of mistakes, their causes and effective approaches to reduce them. In a landmark study from Harvard published in 1991, the investigators scrutinized more than 30,000 charts of patients who had been hospitalized in New York hospitals in order to pinpoint iatrogenic adverse events. They were able to establish that such events were common (3.7%), often associated with negligence (more than a quarter), and that very often they could be prevented [1]. Within less than a decade, the Institute of Medicine (IOM) published its seminal report, estimating that each year up to 98,000 patients die in US hospitals as a result of medical errors which cost dozens of milliards of Dollars and which could be prevented to a large extent [2].

These two studies had a remarkable impact and influence, and were arguably the most prominent of many other publications that led to the creation of "A culture of safety" in health care that was widely adopted in American hospitals as well as worldwide [3-5]. Effective measures targeting monitoring and prevention have been introduced, leading to an ongoing improvement in patient safety and reduction in many types of common iatrogenic harm including errors in patient identification, errors in identification of the organ being treated, prevention of nosocomial infections and falls during hospital admissions, and many more.

However, errors in diagnosis, although included and classified among the negative events mentioned in the IOM report [2], have received relatively little attention over time and their research remains neglected in comparison with the other facets of patient safety. Other aspects have been much more thoroughly targeted which often led to significant 'system' changes and improvements. In contrast, the term "diagnostic error" in PubMed yields only 296 hits in adults in English, and many publications are irrelevant to us as they are limited to a single diagnosis (e.g., infective endocarditis, neck injuries) or specific settings (e.g., emergency department) or to errors in interpretation of a certain diagnostic modality (e.g., biopsies, imaging). The number of papers devoted to the more general field of the formulation of diagnosis, clinical reasoning, the diagnostic cascade and its pitfalls, and errors in diagnosis among unselected ambulatory or admitted patients remains quite limited [6]. Despite their often 'remaining under the radar,' diagnostic errors are common, and their impact on the patient's health outcomes is not only highly significant but amenable to interventions aiming at prevention, improved diagnostic accuracy and increased patient safety.

The forthcoming chapter aims to examine the various types and mechanisms of diagnostic errors, their incidence and unique research methods used in their study, going on to suggest methods of optimal clinical reasoning and diagnosis, applicable for both hospitalized and ambulatory care patients, that may improve the inherently complex diagnostic process and minimize its myriad potential pitfalls.

DEFINITION OF DIAGNOSTIC ERRORS AND RESEARCH METHODOLOGY

A diagnostic error is always defined by an evaluation performed later in the course of the disease. Thus, it is never identified in real time except perhaps for *"delayed diagnosis,"* defined as inappropriately belated diagnosis despite possessing all the information required. Usually, new information obtained *after* the initial diagnosis was made reveals it to be an *"erroneous diagnosis"* that needs to be replaced by another, correct diagnosis. Alternatively, the patient's physicians never reached a diagnosis, a predicament termed *"missed diagnosis"* [7].

The identification and research of diagnostic errors poses many intrinsic difficulties that are hard to overcome. Several different methods of data collection have been used (Table 1), yielding important results and insights, yet none is free of significant weaknesses that make the systematic study of error in medicine especially difficult. For example, discovering major and significant discrepancies between autopsy results and ante-mortem clinical diagnosis is highly important [8-10], but represents extreme conditions, especially as the number of necropsies has shown an unfortunate steep decline worldwide [11]. Relying on recall by physicians or patients through surveys [12, 13] or on voluntary reports [14, 15] must by definition be highly selective and therefore of limited usefulness. So is an analysis of closed malpractice claims [16]. Using case vignettes or simulated standardised patients presenting a clinical problem to clinicians may be illuminating, but suffers from a limited scope and 'artificial' and isolated scenario. The study of trigger events may be more instructive. For example, using all unplanned emergent readmissions to the hospital within 30 days after discharge to identify diagnostic errors in the index admission [17]; or analysing unexpected death/urgent admission after a visit to the primary care physician or discharge from an emergency department [18]. Audits of diagnostic delays for a specific diagnosis (e.g., lung cancer, rheumatoid arthritis, tuberculosis) or audits of specific diagnostic tests interpretation (e.g., mammography, abdominal ultrasound, prostate biopsies) also bring in useful information but remain limited by definition, reflecting an isolated field [19].

Table 1. Diagnostic errors – major sources of information

1. Autopsy data compared to clinical diagnoses
2. Closed malpractice claims
3. Audits of a specific diagnostic modality
4. Case reviews of a specific diagnosis
5. Voluntary reports
   A. Institutional
   B. Reports of errors in diagnosis published in the literature
6. Surveys
   A. Physicians' surveys – recall of errors
   B. Patients' surveys – recall of diagnostic misadventures
7. Workup of 'Scenarios' presented to physicians (or students)
   A. Clinical vignettes
   B. Simulated patients
8. 'Trigger' events
   A. Study of unplanned readmissions ≤30 days post discharge
   B. Retrospective review of Medicare claims after admissions vs. unwarranted recent emergency department discharges
   C. Review of urgent admissions or death soon after a visit to the primary care physician
   D. Analysis of unexpected return visits after an initial primary care "index" visit detected through monitoring of EHRs

INCIDENCE OF DIAGNOSTIC ERRORS

As a result of all these varied research approaches, we know that the widely held presumption that the astounding advances in imaging techniques, endoscopies and laboratory testing have made diagnosis today almost infallible is untrue. Diagnostic errors are definitely not uncommon and their incidence varies considerably according to the setting examined (e.g., hospital vs. primary care) and the research method used (Table 1). Arthur Elstein, a renown psychologist and educator who made substantial contribution to the area of clinical decision making over many years concluded that diagnosis is wrong 10-15% of the time [20, 21]. Importantly, diagnostic errors continue to occur despite the unprecedented improvement in imaging techniques and laboratory testing in recent years and contribute to as many as 70% of medical errors [22]. For example, in a systematic literature review of 42 reported series of autopsies, the median rate of error in diagnosis which was related to the cause of death was 23.5% and in a striking 9% the error contributed to the patient's demise [9]. Another study, notable for the minimal improvement in diagnostic accuracy over decades of technological improvements, identified a disturbing 9% rate of an erroneous diagnosis – believing a non-existent disease to be present, a belief that contributed to the patient's death [8]. Primary care represents a particularly high-risk environment for potential diagnostic errors, as analysed in a recent narrative review [23]. The combination of high volume of patients, time constraints, vast amounts of hidden data in the electronic health record (EHR) and undifferentiated presentations associated with much uncertainty [24] all contribute, endangering patient safety. This is revealed in studies of claims [16] as well as in estimates that cite a 5% of diagnostic errors in the US per year [23]. More focused studies confirm a similarly significant rate in many other countries [25-28]. However, the hospital environment is also a ripe area for the development of diagnostic errors, in particular, high volume of patients/short length of stay (LOS) settings such as emergency departments and departments of general internal medicine.

MECHANISMS AND CLASSIFICATION OF DIAGNOSTIC ERRORS

The landmark study of Mark Graber et al. who analysed in great detail 100 errors in diagnosis among internal medicine patients [7] initiated the currently accepted classification which recognizes three etiological groups of diagnostic errors:

- "No fault" error –
- "System-related" error
- Cognitive error

The first group comprises errors that are practically unavoidable ("no fault") due to a highly unusual presentation of the disease or lack of patient cooperation.

The second group includes a variety of institutional failures ("system-related") that-are primarily responsible for an erroneous diagnosis, such as failing to notice in real time an important laboratory or biopsy result, or lack of review of an imaging or pathology result by a senior clinician, superficial consults, a policy of unreasonably short hospital stays or ambulatory encounters, etc.

The third type, "cognitive errors" occur at the individual clinician-patient interface and lead to a faulty clinical reasoning and thus, errors in decision-making including errors in test ordering and interpretation and errors in the selection of tests and procedures (too few, too many, or the wrong ones selected).

Another classification attempts to determine the stage in the diagnostic process where the error occurred – history, examination, differential diagnosis, test ordering, test interpretation, referrals, follow up, or several of the above acting together. This approach will further classify errors as being related to errors of omission or interpretation, errors related to lack of knowledge base or skills, errors due to overconfidence [29, 30] or inability to handle uncertainty [24], and errors associated with poorly-appreciated contextual factors [31] or implicit bias. Essentially, faulty judgment and not defective knowledge appears to be the predominant mechanism and thus the study of errors in diagnosis is inseparable from that of diagnostic reasoning and decision-making.

An important study analysed 190 instances of diagnostic errors in primary care, identified by EHR monitoring of patients' unexpected return visits after an initial "index" encounter [32]. A total of 68 unique diagnoses out of 190 cases were missed including decompensated congestive failure, serious infectious diseases and cancer. Process breakdowns were seldom patient-related (e.g., patient failed to provide adequate history) or related to diagnostic tests (e.g., erroneous interpretation), follow-up and tracking, or referrals (e.g., appropriate expert is not contacted). Each of these was responsible for approximately 14-19% of contributory factors. In contrast,

¬79% (150/190) were associated with faulty patient-provider encounter – missing important parts of the medical history, faulty physical examination, not ordering the appropriate tests, or failure to review existing medical documents [32]. Patient outcomes were often extremely serious, including very serious harm or permanent damage in 66 cases and mortality in 27. Thus, outpatient practice is also vulnerable to diagnostic errors, which are frequently very dangerous to the patient, but mostly involve common conditions and are liable to preventive interventions. This adds to a previously published systematic review on diagnostic errors in primary care [33]. They do emphasize the need to focus on basic clinical skills (for example, data gathering by history and clinical examination) during the clinical encounter. Potential 'antidotes' and techniques of improving the yield and accuracy of data collection and interpretation will be discussed below.

CLINICAL REASONING AND DIAGNOSTIC ERRORS

No doubt, the analysis of the formulation of diagnosis in the clinician's mind by acquiring, processing and integrating complex data obtained from many sources within a restricted time frame is one of the most intriguing aspects of clinical medicine as well as being highly susceptible to error.

Theoretically, diagnostic problems could be solved by using the Bayes theorem which allows us to determine the probability of disease in a given patient [20]. When using a Bayesian approach, clinicians develop an initial probability that a patient has a disorder. This probability (pre-test probability) is then sequentially revised using information obtained from the history, physical examination, and diagnostic testing to arrive at a final probability estimate (post-test probability). However, this method usually requires complicated calculations using data that is frequently unavailable and therefore it is often impractical [34]. Moreover, clinicians often make mistakes in determinations of both pre-test and post-test probabilities, with resulting significant imprecisions and wide margins of error [35].

Table 2. Important and common biases that may adversely affect the diagnostic process subconsciously, without the physician's awareness

1. Availability bias / Recall bias
The tendency to judge easily recalled possibilities as more likely (a recently-encountered diagnosis, a recently-read paper, diagnoses belonging to the physician's area of expertise)

2. Representativeness bias
The tendency to judge the likelihood of a diagnosis based simply on the similarity of the clinical presentation to an archetype of the disease (although this supposition underlies the principle of 'pattern recognition' it may be a source of error since individual prior probabilities are not taken into account)

3. Anchoring bias
Holding on to the initial diagnostic impression without flexibility despite new conflicting data coming in

4. Confirmation bias
Giving precedence to data that support your own diagnosis while tending to ignore contradictory findings

5. Premature closure
Fixating on an 'established' diagnosis while refusing to consider other viable alternatives or look for further data

6. Framing effect
Clustering together a few pieces of data out of the whole picture to support your diagnosis while disregarding all other non-compatible facts

7. Affective (compassion) bias
A tendency to shift diagnostic judgement due to an emotional involvement (e.g., favouring a benign interpretation of multiple liver lesions when the patient is your friend)

8. Blind obedience bias
Taking for granted or giving undue respect to a higher authority or high-technology-based results despite their being fallible

9. Order effects / Detail effects
The tendency to give more weight to more recent data and more credibility to more detailed (vs. succinct) information

10. Base-rate neglect bias
The tendency to insist on "exotic" unusual impressive diagnoses, despite their rarity

Table 2. (Continued)

11. Uncertainty angst The tendency to perform countless tests in order to rule out even unlikely diagnoses, or diagnoses that have no implication for the patient
12. Implicit contextual biases Age, gender, ethnicity, social status, chronic overriding illness, etc.
13. Overconfidence bias A common tendency to believe that we know more than we do may result in proceeding with incomplete information or failing to consider viable alternatives
14. Diagnostic momentum bias Accepting an existing but wrong diagnostic label without independent criticism

The diagnostic process therefore, is usually based on one of two methods (or both) termed "Pattern recognition" and the "Hypothetico-deductive" method. These are entirely different from one another and indeed, fascinating functional MRI studies have confirmed the two distinct cognitive techniques used by clinicians. When either is being used, a different area in the pre-frontal cortex is activated [36]. The first ("type 1") is intuitive, automatic, rapid (so called, "augenblik" – at the blink of the eye) 'pattern recognition' within seconds which is very effective, more so with time and experience, although it depends on heuristics (mental shortcuts) which are highly prone to distraction by contextual factors and by an array of biases that are often implicated and important to recognize (Table 2) [37, 38]. These insights are based on the Nobel Prize winning (2002) pioneering discoveries of psychologists Amos Tversky and Daniel Kahneman [39] and supported by myriad research data. Basically, the new diagnostic problem is being identified as similar in its essential features to patients we had seen in the past whose diagnosis was well established. Although clinical experience underlies the effective use of the 'pattern recognition' method and results improve over time and are applicable for an increasing number of conditions, it appears to be useful for novices as well [40].

Table 3. The major causes of diagnostic errors**

A. External system factors
  1. Time constraints and overwork affecting quality of data gathering (history taking; clinical examination; review of chart and tests performed) and looking up databases
  2. Missing (or not readily available) significant patient information (diagnoses, tests, imaging)
  3. Deficient alert system notifying physicians of abnormal test results
  4. Common distractions during patient encounters (phones, staff, other patients' demands)
B. Physician's personal factors
  1. Gaps in medical education and CME - faulty knowledge and skills
  2. Attitude - overconfidence, poor ability for teamwork
  3. Emotional well being - fatigue, stress and anxiety, burnout, depression
  4. Physical well-being - illness, medications
C. Pitfalls in data processing - cognitive errors
  1. Poor training in diagnostic reasoning, too few role models
  2. Susceptibility to common heuristics and biases and to contextual non-clinical factors
  3. Lack of full feedback on patients' outcomes - a flat learning curve
  4. Focusing on a single problem at the expense of other important issues (possibly less highlighted)

** A combination of several factors is often to be found at the root of a single diagnostic error. Patient factors or exceedingly rare presentations of disease ('no fault' errors) are non-modifiable and have not been included here.

The other, 'hypothetico-deductive' method ("type 2") is slower, more laborious, elaborate and analytical, usually evaluating 3-5 possible diagnostic alternatives and less prone to error [6]. It involves a rather more laborious evaluation of the probability of each alternative diagnosis in a logical, effort-dependent process and ruling out the less likely entities in the differential diagnosis [36]. In fact, clinicians frequently manipulate between the two approaches to advantage (so called 'dual processing') [7, 39, 41-43] but uncertainty is inherent and susceptibility to error remains so that both type 1 and type 2 processes contribute to errors [42]. Certainly, more complex diagnostic problems are relegated to the 'hypothetico-deductive' approach, whereas simple routine presentations can be dealt with almost automatically. The problem begins when an unusual or multifactorial problem masquerades as a common simple one. It is here that errors may be abundant, often due to multiple operative factors (Table 3). The Table details and distinguishes between external 'organizational' system factors, physicians' personal factors and pitfalls in data processing - cognitive errors. All may predispose to diagnostic errors. These tend to occur concurrently and often, multiple factors (5.9 factors per case in one study) can be identified, with a predominance of cognitive errors [7].

Graber et al. who investigated extensively the origins of cognitive errors in the diagnostic process have classified them into four different facets:

- Deficiencies in knowledge (such as unfamiliarity with a syndrome or wrong interpretation of an electrocardiogram);
- Deficiencies in the acquisition of information (such as skipping important aspects of the history or missing significant signs on examination);
- Faulty processing (such as succumbing to a bias or wrong interpretation of a symptom or sign);
- And deficient verification (such as failure to order an important and specific supporting test or giving priority to an initial diagnosis while ignoring other as likely alternative hypotheses) [7].

Among 100 events studied, there were only 7 "no fault" errors and in the remainder, no less than 548 factors were identified (as mentioned, 5.9/patient) and 320 of them were cognitive factors – much more than faults in knowledge. The most prominent mechanism among them was focusing too early on one conspicuous explanation at the expense of others ("premature closure"). The most frequently recurring errors were those missing a crucial detail in the history or clinical examination; not considering the right diagnosis or considering it too late in the course; and failing to obtain a "revealing" test. Therefore, the pathogenesis of diagnostic errors with the typical cluster of several faults per patient is reminiscent of the "Swiss cheese" model of failures of patient safety and are not solely due to cognitive bias. Analytical approach is also susceptible to error (though to a lesser degree) [44] and physician factors are important contributors (Table 3).

REDUCING ERRORS IN DIAGNOSIS - HOW CAN PATIENT SAFETY BE IMPROVED?

Research on improved quality of clinical reasoning and increased awareness of potential faults in the diagnostic process has still a long way to go [45]. The intricacies of deciphering diagnostic problems and the many implicit pitfalls that the clinicians may unwittingly succumb to are still not even being regularly taught in many faculties of medicine [22, 45]. However, several suggestions regarding the teaching and practice of "low burden of error" medicine can already be made, with emphasis on educational and personal physician measures.

First, rather than frontal lectures, small group bedside exercises led by role models will often yield unexpected diagnoses based on high-quality use of the simple clinical arts [46]. For example, when an experienced attending clinician repeated the basic examination of 100 consecutively admitted patients, 26% had pivotal physical findings (defined by an outcomes adjudication panel as those whose diagnosis and treatment in hospital changed substantially as a result) [47]. This approach is very much in line with internal medicine residents' preferences [48].

Second, the 1992-2016 feature "clinical problem solving" of the New England Journal of Medicine for example [49], provides over 360 highly useful examples of 'rolling' cases and responses of seasoned clinicians to the developing patient script, all explained and analyzed vis-a-vis the final ascertained diagnosis [50]. Their study can lead to a considerably improved insight into an evidence-based diagnostic processing.

Third, habitually verifying the patient's progress and outcomes even (and especially) if the patient has continued his or her care within another health care institution is highly important. Otherwise, the clinician may remain unaware of significant errors and unable to draw conclusions and modify diagnostic process accordingly. For example, several studies have demonstrated that critical test results strongly suggesting the presence of a highly treatable infectious disease (e.g., tuberculosis, HIV) or cancer (e.g., imaging or cytology reports) have been "lost in transition," never came to the attention of the physician who ordered the test or was responsible for the care of the patient, and unfortunately were not acted upon [51-53]. The Emergency Care Research Institute (ECRI) also named diagnostic errors and improper management of test results as the most serious safety challenge in its recent (2019) annual compendium [54]. Organizational [55], but also individual safeguards may annihilate these not uncommon occurrences, deleterious to patient safety.

Fourth, reflexive reflection on the stages and crossroads of the diagnostic process was found to highly valuable for clinicians' professional and personal development. Not only can they verify whether they were right or wrong, but they could also critically review their diagnostic thinking and modify it, incorporating valuable experience gained with each and every clinical encounter [46, 56, 57]. A recent study however, found that among residents reflecting on diagnostic errors in their judgement of simulated cases, reflection by itself provided minimal benefits compared to just knowing the correct answer [58].

Fifth, it is certainly feasible to teach critical thinking skills and instruct students and physicians alike in metacognitive skills with the goal of consciously avoiding biases and improving diagnostic accuracy. However, while there is a total agreement that this should be part of medical education programs, results are mixed at the best and as of today, there is no clear proof that such teaching has a significant impact on the prevention or reduction of diagnostic errors [22]. One eminent group put it even stronger, stating that "educational strategies directed at the recognition of biases are ineffective in reducing errors" [42].

Elstein and Schwartz in their excellent review suggest that two prominent movements in medical education have taken place, leading to a significant improvement in diagnostic thinking [59]. These are problem based learning (PBL) – formulation and testing of varied clinical possibilities starting in the pre-clinical years; and the field of evidence based medicine (EBM) – searching databases for the most suitable patient tailored answer regarding any significant diagnostic or treatment-related problem. In addition, we suggest that a third movement – return to, and adoption of the principle attitudes of humanistic medicine starting in medical school admission requirements and continuing throughout medical education will no doubt enhance future patient-centered care and patient safety as well [56, 60].

Other components putting patients at risk of an erroneous diagnosis are at the institutional (organizational), not the educational level (Table 3). The evidence here is far from conclusive. For example, a 2012 narrative review covering a whole decade (2000-2009) identified 43 articles, but only 6 reported tested interventions and the remainder contained suggestions [61]. Creating a 'culture of safety' in the organization, whether a medical center or primary care, is a target that should be set and promoted, including an audit of diagnostic errors [62, 63]. Tools that have been identified as potentially powerful indicators include facilitating direct reports by physicians and electronic health record (EHR)-based reports detecting process breakdowns in the follow up of abnormal findings [63]. Time constraints are especially important both in the ambulatory care ("The doctor will see you now - for seven minutes...") [64] and for hospitalized patients where increasing costs and a decrease in available beds pushes dangerously down the patient's length of stay (LOS) despite increasing patients' ages and multimorbidity [17, 64-66]. The toll of time constraints grows steadily on, considering the aging of the population worldwide, the increasing complexity of these elderly patients with common multimorbidity [67], the flooding of the busy practitioner with thousands pieces of data buried somewhere in the patient's charts that may in part be vitally important to the diagnostic problem at hand, and the growing number of issues that need to be dealt with to comply with guidelines and the time consuming but obvious need to share information, health literacy and decision making with the patient [68, 69].

Table 4 suggests the seven most important habits ("Commandments") to be personally adopted by clinicians, no matter how time constrained they are, in order to reduce diagnostic errors in their daily encounters with patients. Only the first and fourth approaches will be discussed here, the others to be later addressed in the context of the twenty four principles central to sound clinical reasoning and timely and correct accurate diagnosis.

**Table 4. Seven habits that may reduce diagnostic errors
in either hospitalized or ambulatory patients' care -
The seven 'Commandments'**

First, be systematic and patient-oriented in data collection. Listen to the patient, then proceed in an orderly fashion through the time-honoured elements of the history, examination and review of the tests. With experience and self-training this can be accomplished in minutes and foster avoidance of regrettable omissions. However, slow down when encountering unusual or complex situations.
Second, keep an open mind to alternatives, avoiding 'premature closure,' our most common error. Always ask – what else can it be? Be tuned to any significant, hard to explain deviation from the expected 'script' (or "gestalt") for your diagnosis. And once identified, slow down!
Third, have much respect for the individual patient's pre-test probability (alias: risk factors; alias: susceptibilities). The history of family, occupation, past illness/drugs/procedures, and lifestyle/pet/travel or other relevant exposures - is a frequent harbinger of subsequent illness, even when not apparent at first.
Fourth, look it up: adopt a habit of reflexive consultation with information databases (PubMed, UpToDate, Google) and colleagues. This facilitates a comprehensive differential diagnosis, informed test selection and affords multiple learning opportunities.
Fifth, ensure getting regular feedback on patients' outcomes, comparing them to your own thoughts. When discrepant, reflection begets improvement. Belated test results must be regularly checked and patients followed even when they are no longer under your care.
Sixth, maintain a wide angle – be 'holistic' encompassing all your patient's problems, not just the most glaring complaint.
Seventh, when you don't know, admit it to yourself and to your patient. Honesty is not only the best policy but a strong motivator for increased effort and thoroughness.

A Systematic approach based on observation and listening is always mandatory in avoiding errors. Increasing patients' age and complexity, polypharmacy and flooding of information on tests and hospitalizations threaten to overwhelm busy clinicians making a systematic orderly approach all the more vital today. With constantly increasing options and decreasing of time available in any setting, self-training in proceeding methodically and avoiding errors of omission is a pre-requisite to appropriate decision-making. Keeping to Weed's principles of going from subjective (what the patient and family tell us) to objective (what we find through examination, chest X-ray, ECG and laboratory tests and imaging), and then to assessment and plan – the so called SOAP mnemonic [70], and then creating a problem list for the more complex patients is an excellent starting point. Also, evaluating changes over time and ensuring complete documentation are central. The vast majority of clinical problems are amenable to a systematic application of the traditional clinical tools [71]. A short focused approach can be mastered for simpler problems or time shortage. Still, being systematic, organized and methodical remains crucial in preventing errors. There are few data available on how systematic physicians are in their daily practice. However, skipping important parts of the history and superficial examination seem to be common [72, 73] as is neglecting to look at valuable information already in the patient's charts. As to the patient's examination, the art of clinical observation has become increasingly endangered in recent years. Physicians have become excessively dependent on diagnostic testing [74], and batteries of sophisticated tests are repeatedly applied at the expense of simple observation and more reliance upon basic clinical data, starting with the extended vital signs list (temperature, blood pressure, heart rate, respiratory rate, oxygen saturation, weight, pain scale). Numerous adverse effects ensue including an appalling amount of redundant testing [74, 75], patient harm, prevalent false-positive results, spiralling costs [76] and further atrophy of clinical powers. Observation, implying also attentively listening and getting the patient's agendas, remains a powerful diagnostic tool and the most revealing of all the 4 principles of physical examination – observation, palpation, percussion, and auscultation [47, 77], provided physicians 'know what to look for' and able to use clinical reasoning [72]. Mastering the arts of observation and listening also ensures that clinically-based patient evaluation remains pivotal in daily practice, unlike the prevailing approach.

Accessing databases to weigh multiple possibilities and identify the most appropriate tests for the patient's individual problems is at the core of evidence-based medicine (EBM) and provision of optimal medical care. Consulting databases should be reflexive and routinely used at the point of care to optimize diagnostic (and treatment) decisions and lessen errors [78-81]. Patients will also benefit by avoiding an unnecessary or inappropriate treatment or diagnostic procedure [82]. Moreover, this approach underscores an essential attitude of respect, careful consideration and humility in the physician as well as providing a natural opportunity for continuous learning.

Accessing old patients' charts for past information that may be 'buried' but highly relevant to current problems is also important in avoiding unnecessary tests, understanding the patient's predicament and improving diagnostic decisions. Since new significant clinical research is being published daily and now readily accessible online (including on portable devices) together with up-to-date user-friendly databases, guidelines and textbooks - counting on previous knowledge, anecdotal experience and memory alone is often insufficient. Unfortunately, time constraints and overconfidence often prevail and EBM is still seldom incorporated into daily practice [83], despite its proven practicality [78-81].

In addition, every diagnosis based on 'pattern recognition' had better include a precautionary step of verification in order to identify possible 'unexpected' discordant features and avoid errors. In this step, the essential features of the current patient are being mentally compared with those of the presumptive diagnosis. The two clinical pictures should match, whereas any significant discordance may suggest the need to re-evaluate the 'spot' diagnosis by a more analytical approach. Patients whose cluster of presenting problems is unusual need to be identified as soon as possible. *Slowing down* in these cases and investing more time and effort as appropriate, as well as working with specialist consultants as a team, is bound to increase diagnostic accuracy ("so called "speed – accuracy trade-off") (SAT) [84]. In this context, the 'epidemic' of burnout and fatigue including mental fatigue among physicians [85] adds to proneness to error [86], and possibly, an increase in malpractice claims. Reflexive consultation with renown databases will be highly useful in establishing a selective differential and selection of tests according to their performance characteristics in similar patients (sensitivity, specificity, positive and negative likelihood ratio) [82].

Long-term follow up of the patient after discharge or after being seen in the ambulatory clinic is a very useful habit allowing the physician to become cognizant of any errors that might have occurred and learn from mistakes as well as successes. So is the habit of reflection on the diagnostic process – reflective reasoning [83]. In contrast, reflecting on current diagnostic reasoning to identify potential cognitive biases (so called "Debiasing") appears to be less effective than anticipated since biases occur subconsciously, and the ability to deduce from one case to another is quite limited [41]. Other researchers however, believe differently, and Royce and colleagues have recently suggested that the mixed results in studies of the impact of teaching critical thinking skills may be due to methodological problems [22]. This Harvard group does promote the idea that instruction in metacognitive skills (including awareness of cognitive biases) may well result in improved diagnostic accuracy, enhanced patient safety and better outcomes [22]. Information technology might also be very useful for checking on diagnoses and reducing error, but this field of research is still far from yielding conclusive results. For example, using checklists to present a full differential diagnosis and the major steps in a 'hypothetico – deductive' analysis may prove helpful. This is especially true since a failure to consider the correct diagnosis is among the prominent causes of error [7, 14, 21, 23, 87]. Basically similar checklists are being effectively used in aviation, but diagnostic challenges in medicine appear more heterogeneous, complex and context-dependent. Thus, the potential role of checklists remains controversial [88]. Computerized diagnostic decision support tools are being developed over at least twenty years, but research results on their role in promoting a better and safer diagnosis are not particularly striking [89]. Among them, a basic Google search is the most widely available and may arguably be the most efficient [80]. Simply entering the salient features of the patient's case in a Google search has yielded the correct diagnosis in 58% (95% CI 38-77%) of 26 challenging cases taken out of the case records of the New England Journal of Medicine (excluding management cases) [90]. Among other net-based tools being developed, Isabel has shown especially good results [91]. Others have proposed a short mnemonic-based (CARE) approach to reduce diagnostic errors (Communicate, Assess for biased reasoning, Reconsider differential diagnoses, Enact a plan) [92]. Since there seems to be no agreement on tools or methods to reduce diagnostic errors and enhance patient safety, we suggest following 24 basic suggestions of reaching a valid diagnosis even in difficult cases (Table 5). These will be briefly discussed below.

Table 5. The 24 practical principles of clinical diagnosis*

I. The ABCD Rule – Achieve the most from the Basic Clinical Data
II. Record and arrange key findings using a 'Problem List'
III. Cherchez Les "Red Flags"
IV. Does 'Pattern Recognition' apply? – if so, verify
V. Identify & analyze specific features germane to the case
VI. The Rule of Reflexive Consultation
VII. 'Milk' the Pretest Probability
VIII. Could it be iatrogenic?
IX. Try "Occam's Razor" – the Law of Parsimony
X. The 'Law of Imperfection': prevalent 'Partial' presentations
XI. Is there a tenable Alternative?
XII. The dog that did not bark in the night…
XIII. What is it? Or what it is not!
XIV. Be aware of common biases leading to diagnostic errors
XV. Mind interfering context factors
XVI. Maintain fluidity in clinical reasoning
XVII. Think of "Robbins"
XVIII. Invest Time!
XIX. Consider using the "test of treatment"
XX. Back to step 1?
XXI. If unwell…
XXII. Ensure 'Tracking' & Feedback
XXIII. Avoid "tunnel vision" – be Holistic
XXIV. Respect, show Empathy, Share, Support

* See text. Curiosity is strongly advised [56]. Principles IV and V refer to the two basic (reflexive vs. analytical) methods of reasoning. Principles I VI and XXIII are of prime importance, whereas XXIII and XXIV highlight an essential commitment towards the patient and family that is inseparable from the diagnostic process.

ADOPTING A METHODICAL APPROACH IN ACHIEVING A CORRECT CLINICAL DIAGNOSIS

Diagnosis is the vital engine that carries forward not only the train of treatment but all the patient's health outcomes. Acquiring the science and art of clinical diagnosis is central to medical education, but there is no consensus on how it should be taught and practitioners vary greatly in the techniques they employ for achieving a new diagnosis. Diagnostic problem-solving is highly context-dependent. Thus, it seems disappointing that among internal medicine residents in a major Boston teaching medical center who were asked to state their most valuable recent learning experience, only 8% noted the patient as a participant [48]. Other studies have revealed that patient face time during residency is diminishing. For example, recent studies reveal that internal medicine residents spent only 9%-12% of their time in direct patient care vs. 40%-50% of their time using the computer [93, 94]. Such brief "face time" interactions can hardly suffice and may be associated with deteriorating clinical abilities [95], poor job satisfaction, increased residents' burnout and errors endangering patient safety [86, 96, 97]. In fact, hands-on patient care remains the accepted best, basic, and only way of mastering medicine [98, 99]. Apart from the documented distancing between physicians and their patients, the absence of a single, universal problem-solving process common to all cases and all physicians increases the challenge facing practitioners and educators [56]. Diagnosis is often taught by clinician educators demonstrating it on current patients, but this is usually done without attention to its general principles. Moreover, role model clinicians teaching diagnosis at the bedside [100] have been pronounced 'endangered species' and are hard to come by [101]. CPCs, clinical problem-solving, clinical images and other published 'exercises' in diagnosis provide enlightening examples of clinical reasoning but are often selective, and present unusual patients. Learning from diagnostic errors can be beneficial, whether identified by autopsy studies [8], malpractice claims [16], chart review [7], or self-reported [14]. However, these were studied in retrospect and apply to groups only. Studies of the cognitive aspects of diagnostic decisions based on actual [87] or standardized [83] patients transformed our insight on mechanisms of bias and diagnostic failure, but their practical implications are uncertain. Other studies try to decipher the key to being superior diagnosticians [102, 103] or the essence of medical expertise [104]. However, not many studies address the diagnostic process as a whole, starting from the first patient encounter and data gathering, through analysis and the basic principles of decision-making. Although some excellent books have been devoted to diagnosis, these lengthy texts are not very practical [105, 106]. For example, as mentioned above, the advocated use of Bayesian approach requires complex time-consuming mathematics that most clinicians had rather avoid [107]. We will present an experience- and research-based overview of the major practical principles covering all stages of the diagnostic process which can be used as a framework in teaching, as well as by residents and clinicians in all settings.

The author has been serving as head of a large (400 admissions/month) academic department of medicine for 24 years. Diagnostic principles were derived from a long personal experience in practicing, researching [71] and teaching diagnostic methods to medical students, interns and residents. Commitment to medical education has mandated ongoing follow-up of the literature on decision-making, clinical reasoning and diagnostic errors - an additional important influence on the choice of principles. The author's research in related areas such as the intrinsic value of the history and examination [46, 71], the non-biological aspects of disease [108], the patient-physician relationship [109], clinical excellence [110] and nonclinical influences on decision-making [111] has also been incorporated. Several principles have been included after they proved highly useful in deciphering some intriguing problems in the past [112-118]. Special patient populations have been identified as being especially prone to diagnostic errors. They include patients whose age is younger than expected for the diagnosis, patients who have multiple, interacting morbidities, and patients who cannot effectively communicate their complaints (dementia, depression, culture and language barrier) [18]. Such populations need special attention.

Twenty four principles central to clinical reasoning and diagnosis were identified. Each is briefly described, followed by a comment.

1. The ABCD Rule – Achieve the most from the Basic Clinical Data

Methodical, personal, curiosity-driven [56] gathering of the patient's narrative (all history elements, all potential sources), followed by a systematic (yet problem-directed) examination, often also ECG, chest X-ray and basic laboratory tests will likely diagnose correctly 4 of 5 patients [46, 71] or suggest appropriate investigations. A sound base of knowledge and skills is a prerequisite [47, 102]. Attention to the clinical context and timeframe [118] and to detail, 'The Δ rule' [119], and awareness of the operating characteristics (strengths and limitations) of common history and examination elements [107, 120] are particularly useful. The history (and especially the reason for presentation) remains the most rewarding single source of diagnostic information [113]. Importantly, simple or recurrent problems are often amenable to a much shorter, focused approach.

* Comment. Thoroughness in data collection does not *guarantee* accuracy in interpretation & diagnosis, but remains a strong starting point [20]. In addition, the more patients are seen, the more "illness scripts" are mastered [121], and the more efficient would the next encounter be. Although shunned by some [106], the technique can be applied after some experience within a framework of minutes, retaining its inherent power.

2. Record and arrange key findings using a 'Problem List'

After recording the findings, review the data, identifying meaningful 'clusters' and 'key phrases' and arranging them in a laconic (<~100 words), comprehensive (all types of problems, biologic and psychosocial), dynamic (constantly changing with new information or insight) Problem List [70].

* Comment. Although this step seems to slow you down, it has a high-yield for the provider, ensuring a concise summary of all salient facts, a view of the *whole* picture and an excellent departure for problem-solving, test-selection, presentations and consultations [122]. Here, a first attempt to grasp the gist of patient symptoms and their meaningful connections can be made [123].

3. Cherchez Les "Red Flags"

Screen your problem list giving early consideration to potential 'Red Flags'! Any high impact /high treatability possible diagnoses identified, require urgent intensive attention [116, 117].

* Comment. This is similar to the Rule-Out Worst-case Scenario ('ROWS') principle [88].

4. Does 'Pattern Recognition' apply? – if so, verify

Intuitive, 'augenblick' ('at the blink of the eye') diagnosis suspected by its overall appearance and 'Gestalt' based on *reflexive recognition of resemblance* to previously seen cases, is often rapid (seconds), efficient (effortless) and accurate [41]. However, it is also highly prone to bias and errors (36).

* Comment. Pattern recognition (PR) should be always be tried first but mandates confirmation: a quick verification stage is suggested wherein the provider mentally compares the degree of match between disease characteristics and mental model of the essentials of the suspected diagnosis [121], as if written on 2 overlapping transparencies. Any significant inconsistency may signify error and makes re-evaluation necessary. Reliance on non-analytical reasoning tends to increase with experience but is not limited to experts. Since even accomplished clinicians remain susceptible to bias [83], a further quick "conscious" double-check is always essential [40].

5. Identify & analyze specific features germane to the case

Having failed PR, look for 'specific' features that are both *central* to the case and *unique*. These idiosyncratic clues often allow a shortlist of just a few differential diagnoses [124]. Conditions appearing under 2 or more columns of 'specific' features are especially promising diagnostic possibilities which should be critically evaluated by selecting appropriate tests [114].

* Comment. This variant of the usual analytical ('hypothetico-deductive') (HD) method which names the main etiologies for the patient's presentation (usually, 4 ± 1) following a conscious deliberate search and slowly constructs a workup to rule out/ rule in hypotheses [44], may be more effective. Maintain a skeptic attitude towards previous diagnostic labels, which may, or may not be correct [125].

6. The Rule of Reflexive Consultation

"Look it up" as a habit, as *early* and as *often* as possible using PubMed (even Google), UpToDate, Textbooks, as well as expert colleagues. Main conclusions had better be added to the patient's chart. Such attitude not only ensures a broad comprehensive view but also informed test selection and interpretation [112]; a learning opportunity [46]; and fostering an attitude of humility and maximal care – as opposed to overconfidence [29].

* Comment. This habit also establishes the art of diagnosis as a lifetime learning endeavour [102] and is in line with Graber's "get help" category of interventions likely to reduce diagnostic errors [91].

7. 'Milk' the Pre-test Probability

The diagnosis is very often pathogenetically-related to the patient's past predisposing factors and susceptibilities (genetic, past illnesses, iatrogenic, occupational, lifestyle and other easily ascertainable risk factors and exposures). These predispositions constitute the "pre-test probability," also defined as the expected prevalence of the suspected condition in similar patients.

* Comment. This relationship may be true even when it does not initially seem so. Unfortunately, errors of omission in obtaining these history elements prevail and they may 'surface' only after a long circuitous and costly detour. Thus, a quick but comprehensive survey of predispositions (which may be unapparent at first) had better be given priority, carefully considered [113, 118] and given precedence over "unrelated" conditions arising de novo.

8. Could it be Iatrogenic?

Take a moment to consider the possibility that the patient's medications (possibly OTC or 'natural' preparations) or past medical interventions or procedures underlie the current symptoms, signs or abnormal laboratory tests.

* Comment. This particular brand of 'pre-test probability' is particularly common, comprising the main diagnosis in up to 19% of hospital admissions [126] and a similarly significant proportion of primary care consultations.

9. Try "Occam's Razor" – the Law of Parsimony

Consider the possibility of a single *unifying* diagnosis that may account for all (or most) clinical findings [115], before resorting to multiple concurrent different explanations (so called "Saint's triad") [127].
* Comment. Today's elderly patients with multimorbidity & polypharmacy may easily have more than one operative problem, but still, Occam's law often applies [26].

10. The 'Law of Imperfection': Prevalent 'Partial' Presentations

Do not expect to find a perfect set of symptoms, signs and tests characterizing a given condition in order to make a diagnosis. *Any combination may occur and sometimes even a single symptom and sign may suggest the correct diagnosis.*
* Comment. Complete presentations are most commonly found in textbooks and are *not* necessary for diagnosis.

11. Is there a tenable Alternative?

Finding (or being unable to find) a tenable alternative diagnosis is of paramount importance in the diagnostic considerations.
* Comment. Any 'Key' symptom or sign must be explainable by the diagnosis. A potential alternative explanation detracts, whereas its absence may strongly support it, even in the absence of a typical confirmatory test (few tests are 100% sensitive).

12. The dog that did not bark in the night …

We are all tuned primarily towards positive findings and preoccupied with their importance. However, what is *not* found is often as important –

useful in ruling out diagnoses (by absent key findings) or, even more significant, in drawing attention to an expected but absent feature as a potential specific diagnostic clue.

* Comment. Do not look only at the half-full glass. The empty half may be as revealing and systems as evaluated by examination and found to be normal are highly important in balancing and interpreting the data.

13. What is it? - Or what it is not!

Sometimes it is sufficient (and much more useful) to determine that a given presentation is *not* one of several significant and ominous possibilities. To be able to state its exact cause is occasionally a hard and not cost-effective task (e.g., syncope, headache, low back pain...) [116, 117].

* *Comment. Uncertainty* is the 'bread and butter' of the diagnostic process and a degree of tolerance had better be adopted. This is true provided 'Red Flags' are effectively excluded. Under such circumstances, TIME may be a powerful, safe and frugal diagnostic tool (strategy of 'Watchful Waiting' or the 'test of time'): patients may either get well spontaneously, or the diagnosis will become more obvious [128].

14. Be aware of common Biases leading to diagnostic errors

Several common Cognitive Biases need recognition and attention, since they precipitate pitfalls in diagnosis, especially when using the intuitive pattern recognition mode. Dozens of biases have been identified [129] (Table 2), including: considering recent, memorable, easily recalled diagnoses or those in your field of expertise as more likely ('Availability bias,' 'Recall bias'); preferring data that support it, excluding contradictory material ('Confirmation Bias'; 'Anchoring'); tendency to stop considering alternatives and sticking to your diagnosis ('Premature closure'), tendency to rule out a common disease presenting without its prototypical features ('Representativeness bias'), pursuing rare but more exotic diagnoses ('Base rate neglect bias'); letting emotion influence your reasoning ('affective bias'), and endless testing to exclude even highly unlikely possibilities ('Uncertainty angst').

* Comment. Unfortunately, there is no good evidence that awareness may prevent diagnostic mistakes due to common biases [38]. Nevertheless, until we know more on strategies effective in cognitive debiasing, enhanced reflection on our diagnostic reasoning [88] and critical thinking need to be encouraged.

15. Mind interfering context factors

Contextual factors (such as language barrier, emotional volatility, bias vs. patient characteristics, effect of the encounter setting) are common and may require additional attention so that diagnosis will not be adversely affected [111, 130].

* Comment. Situation-related factors which tend to influence and may skew clinical reasoning process are many and must be recognized and acknowledged.

16. Maintain fluidity in clinical reasoning

For complex problems, remember to examine, reconstruct and reformulate hypotheses as data is obtained and the case evolves.

* Comment. 'Premature closure' remains one of the most common and unyielding errors in diagnosis [7, 122].

17. Think of "Robbins"

Once any *past diagnosis* is encountered, think in terms of the renown pathology textbook: Backwards - What caused it? Forward - What does it cause? And Present - How is it being treated? Can it be linked to the PI (present illness)?

And Think of the complex patient in terms of which *Anatomical systems* are involved (e.g., gastrointestinal tract [GIT], peripheral nervous system

[PNS], myocard) and what *Pathogenetic mechanisms* might apply (e.g., infectious, inflammatory, neoplastic).

* Comment. This type of evaluation is much better than erratic 'name dropping' of many different possible diseases… Both anatomical systems and pathogenetic mechanisms can be further sub-classified (e.g., GIT – small bowel; PNS – autonomic; myocard – diastolic dysfunction; or: Infectious – viral, bacterial, protozoal, etc.). Maintain healthy skepticism: do not take prior diagnoses for granted but take time to briefly check their 'solidity' (validity) [125].

18. Invest Time!

Some diagnostic problems require more effort and are inherently time-consuming. Unless urgent, slow down, consult, reflect, schedule another appointment if necessary [88].
* Comment. Discern as quickly as possible between the straightforward and the complex ('profiling'). The latter will not be deciphered without appropriate *time* allocation and often, *team* work. Complex diagnostic problems are more likely to represent atypical presentation of the more common diseases which should be considered before rare ones.

19. Consider using the "test of treatment"

Failure to respond to treatment as expected may be a clue to diagnostic error. More often, a probable but uncertain single diagnosis may be resolved by 'test of treatment' (e.g., edrophonium in myasthenia; low-dose corticosteroids in polymyalgia rheumatica). Also, clinical deterioration after discontinuation of an empiric treatment may suggest its appropriateness.
* Comment. Provided it is used sparingly and interpreted vs. a pre-determined objective measurement, the 'test of treatment' may be a useful adjunct to diagnosis in selected cases [131].

20. Back to step 1?

In cases where the diagnosis remains obscure despite prolonged and extensive work-up, personally repeating the complete patient's history and examination may point the clinician in the right direction and resolve the difficulty.

* Comment. Rather than repeating sophisticated imaging studies that have already proved non-contributory, going back to the basics with a fresh mind may be more rewarding [113-115].

21. If unwell...

In a 'bad' day (of feeling unwell, fatigued, or burnout) – take extra care or preferably step aside (if you can), for recreation and 'recharge' [132].

* Comment. Persisting despite temporary incapacity is a recipe for mistakes [133].

22. Ensure 'Tracking' & Feedback

Make a habit of regularly obtaining Feedback on your diagnostic performance by comparing your findings and thoughts with test results and 'tracking' your patients' subsequent course. Retain continuous mindfulness and reflection on your performance.

* Comment. Providers often overrate their performance [29, 134, 135]. A habit of tracking and feedback ensures that no abnormal results are disregarded [16] and that mistakes are recognized, encouraging a continuous learning curve, improvement of performance [104] and decrease in future diagnostic errors [136].

23. Avoid "tunnel vision" – be Holistic

Commitment to diagnosis does not end with the patient's primary complaint: heed *any* potential problem that may affect the patient's health in the future [71]. Also, diagnosis does not end with biological disease:

attention to prevalent emotional factors (such as depression, anxiety, stress) may reveal important risk factors and further active diagnoses that require attention [46].

* Comment. Relating to one major condition at the expense of others is a common form of neglect [137-139] and so is disregard of the patient's psychological status, an inseparable and influential feature of illness [46].

24. Respect, show Empathy, Share, Support

The diagnostic process may occasionally be prolonged and creates an ordeal for the patient too. Throughout, be truthful to your patient, even when in doubt or in need to consult a colleague or information source. Once the diagnosis is established and verified, communicate it to the patient/ family without delay, providing information, answering questions – but stressing positive aspects and maintaining hope [109].

* Comment. Sharing and support are essential components of the diagnostic journey and of patient-centered care [60, 140].

In conclusion, diagnostic errors are not uncommon, and are harmful to the patient and costly. They are hard to investigate and their 'pathogenetic' mechanisms are highly varied and very much context-dependent, but their understanding is improving and prevention of many errors is a feasible accomplishment. Thus, preventing diagnostic errors is a highly important facet of increasing patient safety and improving health outcomes, yet empirical studies are scarce and there seems to be little concensus on how it can be done. In this chapter we have emphasized several golden principles of the patient-physician encounter and essentials of reaching a well-founded diagnosis. Being aware of commonly recurring pitfalls in diagnosis is important but following the principles discussed above is useful in every setting and seems a prudent, widely-applicable method of achieving correct diagnosis in a timely fashion, an essential component of enhancing patient safety since diagnostic errors contribute to as many as 70% of medical errors.

REFERENCES

[1] Leape LL, Brennan TA, Laird N, et al. The nature of adverse events in hospitalized patients. Results of the Harvard Medical Practice Study II. *N Engl J Med* 1991; 324:377-84.

[2] Kohn LT, Corrigan JM, Donaldson MS, editors. *To err is human: building a safer health system.* Washington (DC), National Academic Press, 1999.

[3] Weaver SJ, Lubomski LH, Wilson RF, et al. Promoting a culture of safety as a patient safety strategy. A Systematic Review. *Ann Intern Med* 2013; 158: 369–74.

[4] Morello RT, Lowthian JA, Barker AL, et al. Strategies for improving patient safety culture in hospitals: a systematic review. *BMJ Qual Saf* 2013 Jan; 22(1):11-8. doi: 10.1136/bmjqs-2011-000582.

[5] Nieva VF, Sorra J. Safety culture assessment: a tool for improving patient safety in healthcare organizations. *Qual Saf Health Care* 2003; 12(Suppl II):ii17-23.

[6] Graber ML, Wachter RM, Cassel CK. Bringing diagnosis into the quality and safety equations. *JAMA* 2012; 308:1211-2.

[7] Graber ML, Franklin N, Gordon R. Diagnostic errors in internal medicine. *Arch Intern Med* 2005; 165:1493-9.

[8] Kirch W, Schafii C. Misdiagnosis at a university hospital in 4 medical eras. Report on 400 cases. *Medicine* (Baltimore) 1996; 75:29-40.

[9] Shojania KG, Burton EC, McDonald KM, Goldman L. Changes in rates of autopsy-detected diagnostic errors over time. A systematic review. *JAMA* 2003; 289:2849-56.

[10] Sonderegger-Iseli K, Burger S, Muntwyler J, et al. Diagnostic errors in three medical eras: a necropsy study. *Lancet* 2000; 355:2027-31.

[11] Burton JL, Underwood J. Clinical, educational, and epidemiological value of autopsy. *Lancet* 2007; 369:1471-80.

[12] Singh H, Thomas E, Wilson L, et al. Errors in diagnosis in pediatric practice: a multisite survey. *Pediatrics* 2010; 126:70-9.

[13] Blendon RJ, DesRoches CM, Brodie M, et al. Views of practicing physicians and the public on medical errors. *N Engl J Med* 2002; 347:1933-40.
[14] Schiff GD, Hasan O, Kim S, et al. Diagnostic error in medicine. Analysis of 583 physician-reported errors. *Arch Intern Med* 2009; 169:1881-7.
[15] Sevdalis N, Jacklin R, Arora S, et al. Diagnostic error in a national incident reporting system in the UK. *J Eval Clin Pract* 2010; 16:1276-8.
[16] Gandhi TK, Kachalia A, Thomas EJ, et al. Missed and delayed diagnoses in the ambulatory setting: a study of closed malpractice claims. *Ann Intern Med* 2006; 145:488-96.
[17] Balla U, Malnick S, Schattner A. Early readmissions to the department of medicine as a screening tool for monitoring quality of care problems. *Medicine* (Baltimore) 2008; 87:294-300.
[18] Waxman DA, Kanzaria HK, Schriger DL. Unrecognized cardiovascular emergencies among Medicare patients. *JAMA Internal Medicine* 2018; 178:477-84.
[19] Graber ML. The incidence of diagnostic error in medicine. *BMJ Qual Saf* 2013; 22:Suppl II21-II27. doi: 10.1136/bmjqs-2012-001615.
[20] Elstein AS, Schulman LS, Sprafka SA. *Medical problem solving: an analysis of clinical reasoning.* Harvard University Press, Cambridge, Mass., 1978.
[21] Elstein A. Clinical reasoning in medicine. In: Higgs J, Ed. *Clinical reasoning in the health professions*, Oxford, England, Butterworth-Heinemann Ltd, 1995; 49-59.
[22] Royce CS, Hayes MM, Schwartzstein MM. Teaching critical thinking: a case for instruction in cognitive biases to reduce diagnostic errors and improve patient safety. *Acad Med* 2019; 94:187-94.
[23] Singh H, Schiff G, Graber ML, et al. The global burden of diagnostic errors in primary care. *BMJ Qual Saf* 2017; 26:484-94.
[24] Bhise V, Rajan SS, Sittig DF, et al. Defining and Measuring Diagnostic uncertainty in medicine: A systematic review. *J Gen Intern Med* 2017; 33:103-15.

[25] Singh H, Meyer AN, Thomas EJ. The frequency of diagnostic errors in outpatient care: Estimations from three large observational studies involving US adult populations. *BMJ Qual Saf* 2014; 23:727-31.

[26] Khoo EM, Lee WK, Sararaks S, et al. Medical errors in primary care clinics – a cross sectional study. *BMC Fam Pract* 2012; 13:127. doi: 10.1186/1471-2296-13-127.

[27] Bhasale AL, Miller GC, Reid SE, et al. Analysing potential harm in Australian general practice: an incident-monitoring study. *Med J Austral* 1998; 169:73-6.

[28] Sandars J, Esmail A. The frequency and nature of medical errors in primary care: understanding the diversity across studies. *Fam Pract* 2003; 20:231-6.

[29] Berner ES, Graber ML. Overconfidence as a cause of diagnostic error in medicine. Review. *Am J Med* 2008; 121 (5 Suppl):S2-23.

[30] Saposnik G, Redelmeier D, Ruff CC, Tobler PN. Cognitive biases associated with medical decisions: a systematic review. *BMC Med Inform Decis Mak* 2016; 16:138. doi: 10.1186/s12911-016-0377-1.

[31] Ogdie AR, Reilly JB, Pang WG, et al. Seen through their eyes: residents' reflections on the cognitive and contextual components of diagnostic errors in medicine. *Acad Med* 2012; 87:1361-7.

[32] Singh H, Giardina TD, Meyer AND, et al. Types and origins of diagnostic errors in primary care. *JAMA Intern Med* 2013; 173:418-25.

[33] Kostopoulou O, Delaney BC, Munro CW. Diagnostic difficulty and error in primary care – a systematic review. *Fam Pract* 2008; 25:400-13.

[34] Sackett DL, Richardson WS, Rosenberg W, Haynes RB. *Evidence-based medicine: how to practice and teach EBM.* New York, Churchill Livingstone, 1997.

[35] Herrle SR, Corbett EC Jr, Fagan MJ, et al. Bayes' theorem and the physical examination: probability assessment and diagnostic decision-making. *Acad Med* 2011; 86:618-27.

[36] Croskerry P. From mindless to mindful practice – cognitive bias and clinical decision making. *N Engl J Med* 2013; 368:2445-8.

[37] Croskerry P, Nimmo GR. Better clinical decision making and reducing diagnostic error. *J R Coll Physicians Edinb* 2011; 41:155-62.

[38] Croskerry P, Singhal G, Mamede S. Cognitive debiasing 1: origins of bias and theory of debiasing. *BMJ Qual Saf* 2013; 22:ii58-64.

[39] Tversky A, Kahneman D. Judgment under uncertainty: heuristics and biases. *Science* 1974; 185:1124-31.

[40] Ark TK, Brooks LR, Eva KW. Giving learners the best of both worlds: do clinical teachers need to guard against teaching pattern recognition to novices? *Acad Med* 2006; 81:405-9.

[41] Norman G, Eva KW. Diagnostic error and clinical reasoning. *Med Educ* 2010; 44:94-100.

[42] Norman GR, Monteiro SD, Sherbino J, et al. The causes of errors in clinical reasoning: cognitive biases, knowledge deficits, and dual process thinking. *Acad Med* 2017; 92:23-30.

[43] Djulbegovic B, Hozo I, Beckstead J, et al. Dual processing model of medical decision-making. *BMC Med Inform Decis Mak*. 2012 Sep 3;12:94. doi: 10.1186/1472-6947-12-94.

[44] Elstein AS. Thinking about diagnostic thinking: a 30-year perspective. *Adv Health Sci Educ* 2009; 14:7-18.

[45] Mamede S, van Gog T, van den Berge K, et al. Why do doctors make mistakes? A study of the role of salient distracting clinical features. *Acad Med* 2014; 89:114-20.

[46] Schattner A. The clinical encounter revisited. *Am J Med* 2014; 127:268-74.

[47] Reilly BM. Physical examination in the care of medical inpatients: an observational study. *Lancet* 2003; 362:1100-5.

[48] Caton JB, Pelletier SR, Shields HM. Asking what do residents value most: a recent overview of internal medicine residents' learning preferences. *Adv Med Edu Pract* 2018; 9:509-18.

[49] Kassirer JR. Clinical problem-solving--a new feature in the Journal. *N Engl J Med*. 1992; 326:60-1.

[50] Lalazar G, Doviner V, Ben-Chetrit E. Unfolding the diagnosis. Clinical problem-solving. *N Engl J Med* 2014; 370:1344-8.

[51] Ghandi TK. Fumbled handoffs: one dropped ball after another. *Ann Intern Med* 2005; 142:352-8.

[52] Dahm MR, Georgiou A, Westbrook JI, et al. Delivering safe and effective test-result communication, management and follow-up: a mixed-methods study protocol. *BMJ Open* 2018; Feb 15; 8(2):e020235. doi: 10.1136/bmjopen-2017-020235.

[53] Callen JL, Westbrook JI, Georgiou A, Li J. Failure to follow-up test results for ambulatory patients: a systematic review. *J Gen Intern Med.* 2012; 27:1334-48.

[54] ECRI Institute. *Top 10 Patient Safety Concerns for 2019.* https://www.ecri.org/landing-top-10-patient-safety-concerns-2019.

[55] Lacson R, Prevedello LM, Andriole KP, et al. Four-year impact of an alert notification system on closed-loop communication of critical test results. *AJR Am J Roentgenol* 2014; 203:933-8.

[56] Schattner A. Curiosity. Are you curious enough to read on? Editorial. *J Royal Soc Med* 2015; 108:160-4.

[57] Mamede S, van Gog T, Moura AS, et al. Reflection as a strategy to foster medical students' acquisition of diagnostic competence. *Med Educ* 2012; 46:464-72.

[58] Monteiro SD, Sherbino J, Patel A, et al. Reflecting on Diagnostic Errors: Taking a Second Look is Not Enough. *J Gen Intern Med* 2015; 30:1270–4.

[59] Elstein AS, Schwarz A. Clinical problem solving and diagnostic decision making: selective review of the cognitive literature. *BMJ 2002*; 324:729-32.

[60] Schattner A. The essence of humanistic medicine. *QJM 2020*; 113:3-4.

[61] Singh H, Graber ML, Kissam SM, et al. System related interventions to reduce diagnostic error: a narrative review. *BMJ Qual Saf* 2012; 21:160-70.

[62] Alsalem G, Bowie P, Morrison J. Assessing safety climate in acute hospital settings: a systematic review of the adequacy of the psychometric properties of survey measurement tools. *Health Serv Res* 2018; 18:353.

[63] Graber ML, Trowbridge R, Myers JS, et al. The next organizational challenge: finding and addressing diagnostic error. *J Comm J Qual Patient Saf* 2014; 40:102-10.

[64] Salgo P. The doctor will see you for exactly seven minutes. *The New York Times* 2006; March 22.

[65] Konrad TR, Link CL, Shackelton RJ, et al. It's about time: physicians' perceptions of time constraints in primary care medical practice in three national healthcare systems. *Med Care* 2010; 48:95-100.

[66] Tran HV, Lessard D, Tisminetzky MS, et al. Trends in length of hospital stay and the impact on prognosis of early discharge after a first uncomplicated acute myocardial infarction. *Am J Cardiol* 2018; 121:397-402.

[67] Salisbury C, Man MS, Bower P, et al. Management of multimorbidity using a patient-centred care model: a pragmatic cluster-randomised trial of the 3D approach. *Lancet* 2018; 392:41-50.

[68] Schattner A, Rudin D, Jellin N. Good physicians from the perspective of their patients. *BMC Health Serv Res* 2004; 4:26.

[69] Schattner A. Patient care outside of office visits. *J Gen Intern Med* 2011; 26:234.

[70] Weed LL. Medical records that guide and teach. *N Engl J Med* 1968; 278:593-600.

[71] Paley L, Zornitzki T, Cohen J, Friedman J, Kozak N, Schattner A. Utility of clinical examination in the diagnosis of emergency department patients admitted to the department of medicine of an academic hospital. *Arch Intern Med* 2011; 171:1394-6.

[72] Feddock CA. The lost art of clinical skills. *Am J Med* 2007; 120:374-8.

[73] Duke M. Whither the history and physical? *Conn Med* 2008; 72:611-2.

[74] Schattner A. The unbearable lightness of diagnostic testing: time to contain inappropriate test ordering. *Postgrad Med J* 2008; 84:618-21.

[75] Brenner DJ. Medical imaging in the 21st Century – getting the best bang for the rad. *N Engl J Med* 2010; 362:943-5.

[76] Neilson EG, Johnson KB, Rosenbloom ST, Dupont WD, Talbert D, Giuse DA, et al. The impact of peer management on test-ordering behavior. *Ann Intern Med* 2004; 141:196-204.

[77] Orient JM. *Sapira's art & science of bedside diagnosis*. Wolters Kluwer/Williams & Wilkins, Philadelphia, 2010.

[78] Sackett DL, Straus SE. Finding and applying evidence during clinical rounds. The "evidence cart." *JAMA* 1998; 280:1336-8.

[79] Hoogendam A, Stalenhoef AF, Robbe PF, Overbeke AJ. Answers to questions posed during daily patient care are more likely to be answered by UpToDate than PubMed. *J Med Internet Res* 2008; 10:e29. doi: 10.2196/jmir.1012.

[80] Schattner A, Abel N, von der Walde J. Doctor Google, Mister PubMed? *Neth J Med* 2013; 71:166.

[81] Goodman K, Grad R, Pluye P, et al. Impact of knowledge resources linked to an electronic health record on frequency of unnecessary tests and treatments. *J Contin Educ Health Prof* 2012; 32:108-15.

[82] Halkin A, Reichman J, Schwaber M, et al. Likelihood ratios: getting diagnostic testing into perspective. *QJM* 1998; 91:247-58.

[83] Mamede S, van Gog T, van den Berge K, et al. Effect of availability bias and reflective reasoning on diagnostic accuracy among internal medicine residents. *JAMA* 2010; 304:1198-203.

[84] Spieser L, Servant M, Hasbroucq T, Burle B. Beyond decision! Motor contribution to speed-accuracy trade-off in decision-making. *Psychon Bull Rev* 2017; 24:950-6.

[85] Rotenstein LS, Torre M, Ramos MA, et al. Prevalence of burnout among physicians: a systematic review. *JAMA* 2018; 320:1131-50.

[86] West CP, Tan AD, Habermann TM, Sloan JA, Shanafelt TD. Association of resident fatigue and distress with perceived medical errors. *JAMA*. 2009; 302:1294-300.

[87] Vickrey BG, Samuels MA, Ropper AH. How neurologists think. A cognitive psychology perspective on missed diagnoses. *Ann Neurol* 2010; 67:425-33.

[88] Ely JW, Graber ML, Croskerry P. Checklists to reduce diagnostic errors. *Acad Med* 2011; 86:307-13.

[89] Graber ML, Mathew A. Performance of a web-based clinical diagnosis support system for internists. *J Gen Intern Med*, 2008; 23 (Suppl 1):37-40.

[90] Tang H, Kwoon JH Ng. Googling for a diagnosis—use of Google as a diagnostic aid: internet based study. *BMJ* 2006; 333:1143-5.

[91] Graber ML, Kissam S, Payne VL et al. Cognitive interventions to reduce diagnostic error: a narrative review. *BMJ Qual Saf*, 2012; 21:535-57.

[92] Rush JL, Helms SE, Mostow EN. The CARE approach to reducing diagnostic errors. *Int J Dermatol* 2017; 56:669-73.

[93] Block L, Habicht R, Wu AW, et al. In the wake of the 2003 and 2011 duty hours regulations, how do internal medicine interns spend their time? *J Gen Intern Med* 2013; 28:1042-7.

[94] Mamykina L, Vawdrey DK, Hripcsack G. How do residents spend their shift time? A time and motion study with a particular focus on the use of computers. *Acad Med* 2016; 91:827-32.

[95] Mangione S, Nieman LZ. Cardiac auscultatory skills of inernal medicine and family practice trainees. A comparison of diagnostic proficiency. *JAMA* 1997; 278:717-22.

[96] West CP, Huschka MM, Novotny PJ, et al. Association of perceived medical errors with resident distress and empathy: a prospective longitudinal study. *JAMA* 2006; 296:1071–8.

[97] Block L, Wu AW, Feldman L, Yeh HC, Desai S. Residency schedule, burnout and patient care among first-year residents. *Postgrad Med J* 2013; 89:495-500.

[98] Stickrath C, Noble M, Prochazka A, et al. Attending rounds in the current era: what is and is not happening. *JAMA Intern Med* 2013; 173:1084-9.

[99] Berwick DM. What 'patient-centered' should mean: confessions of an extremist. *Health Aff* (Millwood) 2009; 28:w555-65.

[100] Cruess SR, Cruess RL, Steinert Y. Role modelling – making the most of a powerful teaching strategy. *BMJ* 2008; 336:718-21.

[101] LaCombe MA. On bedside teaching. *Ann Intern Med* 1997; 126:217-20.

[102] Mylopoulos M, Lohfeld L, Norman G, et al. Renowed physicians perceptions of expert diagnostic practice. *Acad Med* 2012; 87:1413-7.
[103] Mylopoulos M, Regehr G. Cognitive metaphors of expertise and knowledge: prospects and limitations for medical education. *Med Edu* 2007; 41:1159-65.
[104] Ericsson KA. An expert-performance perspective of research on medical expertise: the study of clinical performance. *Med Edu* 2007; 41:1124-30.
[105] Kassirer JP, Kopelman RI. *Learning clinical reasoning.* Williams & Wilkins, Baltimore, 1991,
[106] Sackett DL, Haynes RB, Guyatt GH, Tugwell P. *Clinical epidemiology. A basic science for clinical medicine.* Little Brown, Boston, 1991, pp. 1-170.
[107] Grimes DA, Schulz KF. Refining clinical diagnosis with likelihood ratios. *Lancet* 2005; 1500-5.
[108] Schattner A. The emotional dimension and the biological paradigm of illness – time for a change. *Quart J Med* (Oxford) 2003; 96:617-21.
[109] Schattner A. The silent dimension. Expressing humanism in each medical encounter. *Arch Intern Med* 2009; 169:1095-9.
[110] Schattner A. Being Better Clinicians: an Acronym to Excellence. *Quart J Med* (Oxford) 2013; 106:385-8.
[111] Schattner A. Are physicians' decisions affected by multiple nonclinical factors? *Internal Medicine: Open* 2014; 4:152. doi:10.4172/2165-8048.1000152.
[112] Schattner A, Gabovich N, Lifschiz A, Becker S. Medline solution. *Lancet* 1999; 353:462.
[113] Schattner A, Zimhony O, Avidor B, Giladi M. Asking the right question. *Lancet* 2003; 361:1786.
[114] Schattner A, Zornitzki T. When the whole-body scan shows no abnormality. *Lancet* 2007; 369:2214.
[115] Schattner A. As sharp as Occam? *Lancet* 2009; 373:1996.
[116] Schattner a, Meital A, Mavor E. Red-flag syncope: spontaneous splenic rupture. *Am J Med* 2014; 127:501-2.

[117] Schattner A, Meital A, Ben-Galim P. Low back pain, lassitude and loss of appetite. *J Royal Soc Med Open* 2014; 5.
[118] Schattner A. Unusual venous thrombosis in a 35-year-old man. *CMAJ* 2014; 186:51-5.
[119] Schattner A. Determining the 'point of change' in the patient's history-the delta rule. *Int J Med Edu* 2015; 6:63-4.
[120] Simel DL, Rennie D. Eds. The Rational Clinical Examination. Evidence-based clinical diagnosis. *JAMA & Archives Journal*, McGraw Hill, New York 2009.
[121] Schmidt HG, Rikers RMJP. How expertise develops in medicine: knowledge encapsulation and illness script formation. *Med Edu* 2007; 41:1133-9.
[122] Institute of Medicine (US). Committee on Improving the Patient Record. In: *The computer-based patient record: an essential technology for health care*. Dick RS, Steen EB, Detmer DE, Eds. National Academy Press, Washington DC, 1997.
[123] Lloyd FJ, Renya VF. Clinical gist and medical education. Connecting the dots. *JAMA* 2009; 302:1332-3.
[124] Eco U. Horns, hooves, insteps. In: Eco U, Sebock TA (eds.) *Dupin, Holmes, Peirce. The sign of three*. Indiana University Press, Indianapolis, 1988, pp. 198-220.
[125] Ilgen JS, Eva KW, Regehr G. What's in a label? Is diagnosis the start or the end of clinical reasoning? *J Gen Intern Med* 2016; 31:435-7.
[126] Atiqi R, van Bommel E, Cleophas TJ, Zwinderman AH. Prevalence of iatrogenic admissions to the departments of medicine/cardiology/ pulmonology in a 1250 bed general hospital. *Int J Clin Pharmacol* 2010; 48:517-24.
[127] Hilliard AA, Weinberger SE, Tierney LM, et al. Clinical problem-solving. Occam's razor versus Saint's triad. *N Engl J Med* 2004; 350:599-603.
[128] Heneghan C, Glasziou P, Thompson M, et al. *Diagnostic strategies used in primary care*. BMJ 2009; 338:b946.

[129] Mull N, Reilly JB, Myers JS. An elderly woman with 'heart failure': cognitive biases and diagnostic error. *Cleve Clin J Med* 2015; 82:745-53.

[130] Durning S, Artino AR, Pangaro L, et al. Context and clinical reasoning: understanding the perspective of the expert's voice. *Med Edu* 2011; 45:927-38.

[131] Glasziou P, Rose P, Heneghan C, Balla J. Diagnosis using "test of treatment." *BMJ* 2009; 338:b1312.

[132] Balch CM, Shanafelt T. Combating stress and burnout in surgical practice: a review. *Adv Surg* 2010; 44:29-47.

[133] Firth-Cozens J, Greenhalgh J. Doctors' perceptions of the links between stress and lowered clinical care. *Soc Sci Med* 1997; 44:1017-22.

[134] Montano DE, Phillips WR. Cancer screening by primary care physicians: a comparison of rates obtained from physician self-report, patient survey, and chart audit. *Am J Public Health* 1995; 85:795-800.

[135] Jenner EA, Fletcher B, Watson P, et al. Discrepancy between self-reported and observed hand hygiene behaviour in healthcare professionals. *J Hosp Inf* 2006; 63:418-22.

[136] Schiff GD. Minimizing diagnostic error: the importance of follow-up and feedback. *Am J Med* 2008; 121 (5 Suppl):S38-42.

[137] Redelmeier DA, Tan SH, Booth GL. The treatment of unrelated disorders in patients with chronic medical diseases. *N Engl J Med* 1998; 338:1516-20.

[138] Dexter PR, Perkins S, Overhage M, et al. A computerized reminder system to increase the use of preventive care for hospitalized patients. *N Engl J Med* 2001; 345:965-70.

[139] Spinewine A, Swine C, Dhillon S, et al. Appropriateness of use of medicines in elderly inpatients: qualitative study. *BMJ* 2005; 331:935.

[140] Epstein RM, Fiscella K, Lesser CS, Stange KC. Why the nation needs a policy push on patient-centered health care. *Health Aff* (Millwood) 2010; 29:1489-95.

In: Investigating Patient Safety
Editor: Gloria Hale
ISBN: 978-1-53617-344-4
© 2020 Nova Science Publishers, Inc.

Chapter 3

THE IMPLEMENTATION OF THE COMMON ASSESSMENT FRAMEWORK IN PUBLIC HEALTHCARE ORGANIZATIONS: IMPROVING PATIENT SAFETY THROUGH IMPROVEMENT OF ORGANIZATIONAL PERFORMANCE

Stella Korouli[1]*, MSc, Vasiliki Kapaki[2], PhD and Adamantia Englezopoulou[3], PhD(c)
[1]Medical School, National and Kapodistrian University of Athens, Athens, Greece
[2]School of Social and Political Sciences, University of Peloponnese, Corinth, Greece
[3]Laiko General Hospital of Athens, Athens, Greece

---

* Corresponding Author's Email: stellkor@gmail.com

ABSTRACT

The Common Assessment Framework (CAF) constitutes a holistic analysis of the performance of one organization, approaching it from different perspectives simultaneously. According to this, the excellent results for the organizational performance, citizens/customers and society rely on leadership, planning/design, human resources, partnerships, resources, as well as administrative processes. CAF is based on 8 basic principles, the so called "Excellence Principles", namely Results orientation, Focus on citizen/customer, Leadership and Consistency of aim, Management through processes and facts, Development and participation of human resources, Continuous learning, Innovation and improvement, Development of partnerships and Corporate social responsibility. These principles have been incorporated in the CAF structure through 9 criteria, which are further analyzed in 28 subcriteria. Each of the principles has 4 maturity levels, which define over time the course of one organization towards excellence. The CAF 9 criteria represent the main aspects that need to be taken into consideration during the analysis of any organization. These are categorized in 5 criteria-enablers, which cover what the organization does (Leadership, Strategy & Planning, Human Resources, Partnerships & Resources and Processes) and 4 criteria- results, which cover what the organization achieves (Citizens/Customers oriented results, Human Resources oriented results, Society oriented results and Key performance results). By conducting a self-assessment Public Organizations may define in their function their strengths, as well as areas for improvement. The self-assessment process is guided by a specific rating system. The CAF implementation is a continuous process, as the conclusions from one assessment should lead to a plan with improvement actions, which, after their implementaion, should be re-assessed using the CAF, so to achieve continuous administrative improvement. As a conclusion, the CAF is a Total Quality Management (TQM) tool that Public Organizations can use for free for their self-assessment, aiming at improving their administrative capacity and services, without having to ask for support from external sources.

Keywords: self-assessment of hospital, common assessment framework, quality in healthcare services

INTRODUCTION

The CAF belongs to the TQM tools and in Europe it is used for free as of year 2000 to assist Public Organizations in using TQM techniques in a simple way so that they can improve their administrative capacity and the services provided to citizens and other enterprises.

The CAF constitutes a holistic analysis of one organization, approaching it from different perspectives simultaneously and assessing the results achieved, either by its entirety or by its different divisions, in terms of organizational performance, citizens'/customers' satisfaction and society's satisfaction (EIPA, 2019). By being common for Organizations of the Public Sector, it ensures comparability of results among similar services.

European Public Administration Network (EUPAN) introduced this tool on the principles and philosophy of TQM and Public Management. The CAF is available for free and it is inspired by the European Foundation for Quality Management (EFQM) model, sharing the same 9 criteria. According to fundamental European guidance, all processes of Public Organizations must be part of a quality system, therefore, the implementation of the CAF, in addition to the use of other systems and quality tools, is a topic of first priority for the administrative transformation and the improvement of the Public Sector.

The essence of the CAF use is the continuous administrative improvement through appropriately designed actions or measures. The CAF constitutes a complete study of the structure and function of one Public Organization at a defined point of time. The process of self-assessment is based on real facts and evidence-based views for each criterion/subcriterion. The employees of the organization can perform the assessment themselves, without support from external partners.

The implementation of the CAF is a continuous process, since the results from one assessment should lead to the compilation of a plan with improvement actions, which, after their implementation, are re-assessed based on the same tool, in order to achieve continuous administrative improvement.

Public Organizations can implement the CAF either in their entirety or in specific divisions, yet always as a single tool and never in fragments, with the selective use of specific criteria and subcriteria.

ORIGIN AND DEVELOPMENT OF THE CAF

Public Administration throughout Europe, more than ever in our days, is asked by society to prove and improve the value it brings as far as the maintenance and further development of the societal well-being are concerned. In times of socio-financial austerity, the effectiveness of the public policies, the organizational adequacy and the quality of public services constitute factors of vital importance, which define the response to the changing needs and expectations of citizens and enterprises (Dimitriou and Archontas, 2015).

In the countries-members of the European Union, Public Administration is trying to meet all these societal requirements and has undertaken many initiatives for the implementation of new techniques and methods, aiming at improving its effectiveness, performance, as well as its financial and societal responsibility. To this direction different approaches have taken place in all types of Public Organizations and sectors of public responsibility, at European, national, federal, regional and local level. One of the key factors that affected the results of these initiatives was the lack of a coherent and sustainable approach (Michalopoulos, Polykratis and Dimitriou, 2017).

In 1998 from discussion among the General Managers of Public Administration of countries-members within EUPAN, the need for a common European quality framework arose, to be used across the Public Sector as a self-assessment tool. It was, therefore, decided that this quality framework be jointly developed under the auspices of the Innovative Public Services Group (IPSG), an unofficial working group from experts at national level, established by General Managers of EUPAN.

The first CAF edition was created in 1998 and 1999 from IPSG with the support of EFQM, Speyer Academy and the European Institute of Public Administration (EIPA). Speyer Academy had established the homonymous quality award for the Public Sector in German speaking European countries (Engel, 2002).

The CAF standard was implemented in 2000 during the 1st European Quality Conference in Lisbon. In 2001 in Maastricht, Netherlands the European CAF Resource Center was established in EIPA, as a center of specialization for the CAF implementation with the aim to train, consult and support countries members of the European Union in promoting and further enhancing the CAF.

The first two years of the implementation of CAF were evaluated by a study on its use. The results of the study led to the improved CAF 2002 edition, presented at the 2nd European Quality Conference in Denmark. A further study on the CAF use in 2005 indicated a number of areas requiring further improvement. Such improvements were the increase of the coherence and the simplification of the tool, the increase of user-friendliness with the elaboration of examples and special vocabulary, the development of a better scoring system for specific users and the incorporation of guidance documents about benchlearning. Therefore, the CAF was improved for the second time in 2006 and its new edition, the CAF 2006 edition, was presented at the 4th European Quality Conference in Finland. In 2009 and 2010 the establishment of a process of external feedback on the CAF use followed, along with a special edition for the teaching sector, respectively (Staes et al., 2011).

The most recent edition of CAF is this of year 2013, with the incorporation of changes that arose from observations collected from 400 users of the tool and its national correspondents in the countries-members of the European Union. With this revision, the tool improved significantly, with aim the benefit of all stakeholders of the Public Sector in general and more specifically of citizens (Michalopoulos, Polykratis and Dimitriou, 2017). For example, concepts like the users' orientation, public performance, innovation, ethics, effective collaboration with other organizations and social responsibility have been developed in depth, creating new possibilities for further development of the Public Sector organizations (Dimitriou and Archontas, 2015) (Table 1).

Table 1. The development of CAF

Year	Event
1998	Agreement on the development of the CAF within EUPAN
2000	CAF Implementation
2001	Foundation of European CAF Resource Center in EIPA Institute (Maastricht, Netherlands)
2002	First revision of the standard: Implementation of CAF 2002 edition
2006	Second revision of the standard: Implementation of CAF 2006 edition
2009	Implementation of external feedback process
2010	CAF edition specialized for teaching sector
2013	Third revision of the standard: Implementation of CAF 2013 edition

As far as the adoption of the tool is concerned, 59 European countries have currently implemented the CAF, having in total 3.989 registered users (EIPA, 2019).

OBJECTIVE OF THE CAF STANDARD

The CAF can act as a catalyst for an integrated improvement process within one Public Organization and has five basic objectives (EIPA, 2019) (Dimitriou and Archontas, 2015):

- To introduce Public Organizations in the excellence culture and the TQM principles,
- To guide them gradually to an integrated quality cycle, which consists of the Deming Cycle stages,
- To enable the self-assessment of one Public Organization and support it in diagnosing improvement areas and taking the appropriate actions,
- To act as a bridge between the different standards used for quality management in both Public and Private Sectors &
- To enable the bench learning among different organizations of the Public Sector

The organizations that implement the CAF are aspired to achieve excellent performance. The effective use of the CAF should lead to further development of this culture of excellence within the organization in a short time period.

STRUCTURE OF THE CAF STANDARD

According to the CAF, the excellent results in terms of organizational performance, citizens/customers' satisfaction and society's satisfaction depend on leadership, planning/design, human resources, partnerships, resources, as well as administrative processes.

The CAF is based on 8 basic principles, the so called "Excellence Principles". These principles make the difference between traditional, bureaucratic, Public Organizations and Public Organizations oriented towards Total Quality (Dimitriou and Archontas, 2015).

These principles are the following (Dimitriou and Archontas, 2015) (EIPA, 2019):

1. *Orientation towards results:*
   The organization focuses on results, for the benefit of all interested parties (Public Authorities, citizens/customers, partners and human resources of the organization) in conjunction with the objectives set.
2. *Focus on citizen/customer:*
   The organization focuses on the needs of both current and potential citizens/customers, promoting their active participation in the development of its products and services and the improvement of its performance.
3. *Leadership and consistency of purpose:*
   This principle combines leadership that has vision and inspiration with purpose, which remains consistent in a changing environment. The leadership clearly establishes the mission, vision and values. In addition, it creates and maintains an internal

environment in which human resources have the possibility to participate fully to meet the objectives of the organization.

4. *Management through processes and facts:*
    The desired outcome comes successfully when relevant resources are managed as process and the effective decisions are driven by the analysis of facts and information.

5. *Development and participation of human resources:*
    Human resources at all levels constitute the essence of the organization. The full participation of employees allows the use of their skills for the benefit of the organization. The personnel's contribution should be maximized through their development and participation, as well as through the creation of a working environment of common values, trust, transparency, empowerment and recognition.

6. *Continuous learning, innovation and improvement:*
    The excellence constitutes a challenge for the current status and activates change through continuous learning. Therefore, continuous improvement should constitute a permanent objective of the organization.

7. *Development of partnerships*:
    The organizations of the Public Sector need other Public Organizations to meet their objectives. Consequently, they should develop and maintain partnerships that add value, through a relationship of interdependence.

8. *Corporate social responsibility:*
    Public Organizations must own their part of social responsibility. This means that they must respect ecological sustainability and try to meet the high expectations and requirements of the local and international community.

The CAF standard incorporates in its structure the Excellence Principles. Each of the principles is consisted by 4 maturity levels. The organization will reach these levels gradually during its course towards excellence through an integrated Quality Cycle, (Deming Cycle/Plan- Do- Check- Act, PDCA) (Figure 1).

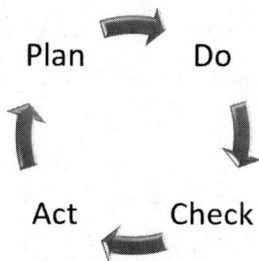

Source: Encyclopedia of Production and Manufacturing Management, 2000.

Figure 1. The Deming Plan, Do, Check, Action (PDCA) Cycle.

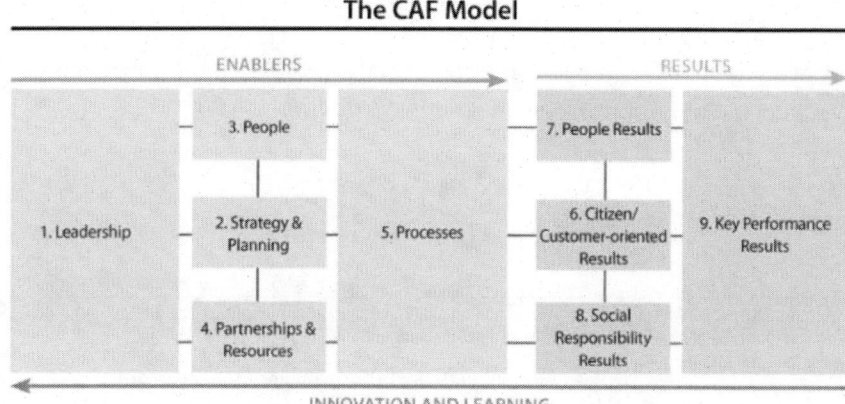

Source: Dimitriou and Archontas, 2015.

Figure 2. The CAF Model.

The CAF has 9 criteria that represent the key aspects that need to be taken into account in the analysis of any organization. There are 5 criteria-enablers (Leadership, Strategy & Planning, Human Resources, Partnerships & Resources and Processes) and criteria-results (Results oriented to Citizen/Customer, Results oriented to Human Resources, Results oriented to Society and Key Performance Results) (EIPA, 2019). The criteria-enablers cover what the organization does, while the criteria-results cover what the organization achieves. With the conduct of a self-assessment, the Public

Organizations can identify in their function, as well as in their aspiration for desired results, areas for improvement (Tomazevic, Seljak and Aristovnik, 2014) (Figure 2).

The 9 criteria of the standard are further analyzed in 28 subcriteria, which identify the main issues that need to be addressed when a Public Organization is assessed. Each of these subcriteria comprises a series of examples (EIPA, 2019). These examples reflect a large number of successful practices across Europe. Despite the fact that not all criteria are applicable to all organizations, many of these require special attention during the self-assessment. The incorporation of the conclusions from the assessment of the criteria-enablers and the criteria-results into the administrative practices constitutes the never-ending cycle of innovation and learning, which accompanies organizations on their way to excellence (Dimitriou and Archontas, 2015).

Each organization can adjust freely the CAF to its specific conditions or even exceptional circumstances, yet with all 9 criteria and 28 subcriteria, as presented in Table 2:

Table 2. The CAF criteria

1st Criterion: Leadership	It assesses the way with which people at the helm and managers shape the mission of one Public Organization (P.O.), facilitate its fulfillment and contribute to the realization of the vision. It includes 4 sub-criteria.
Sub-criterion 1.1	The Leadership provides one clear direction of the P.O., developing vision, mission and values.
Sub-criterion 1.2	What the Leadership does to develop and implement a performance management system and changes.
Sub-criterion 1.3	What the Leadership does to encourage, support employees and act as a role model.
Sub-criterion 1.4	How the Leadership manages the relations with the politicians and the rest groups of interest to ensure common responsibilities.
2nd Criterion: Strategy & Planning	It assesses the way the P.O. implement its mission through one specific strategy oriented towards the groups of interest and with the support of public policies, programs, processes, etc. It includes 4 sub-criteria.

Sub-criterion 2.1	What the P.O. does to collect information regarding the current or future needs of the parties involved in its function.
Sub-criterion 2.2	What the P.O. does to develop, revise and update its strategy and planning taking into consideration the needs of all the involved parties in its function and the available resources.
Sub-criterion 2.3	What the P.O. does to implement strategy and planning throughout the organization.
Sub-criterion 2.4	What the P.O. does to design, implement and update its program for modernization and innovation.
3rd Criterion: Human Resources Management	It assesses the way a P.O. manages and develops the knowledge and skills of its personnel. It includes 3 sub-criteria.
Sub-criterion 3.1	What the P.O. does to program, manage and improve human resources with transparency in relation to its strategy and planning.
Sub-criterion 3.2	What the P.O. does to determine, develop and make use of employees' capabilities, harmonizing individual objectives with organizational ones.
Sub-criterion 3.3	What the P.O. does to involve employees by developing open dialogue and empowering them, supporting their well-being.
4th Criterion: Partnerships & Resources	It assesses the way the P.O. designs and manages the external relationships and the internal resources in order to support its policy, strategy and the effective function of its processes. It includes 6 sub-criteria.
Sub-criterion 4.1	What the P.O. does to develop and implement basic relationships of partnerships.
Sub-criterion 4.2	What the P.O. does to develop and implement partnerships with citizens/customers.
Sub-criterion 4.3	What the P.O. does to manage finances.
Sub-criterion 4.4	What the P.O. does to manage information and knowledge.
Sub-criterion 4.5	What the P.O. does to manage technology.
Sub-criterion 4.6	What the P.O. does to manage its facilities.
5th Criterion: Management of Processes & Changes	It assesses the way the P.O. manages and improves the processes in order to support its strategy and satisfy its citizens/customers.

Table 2. (Continued)

Sub-criterion 5.1	What the P.O. does to determine, design and continuously improve its processes.
Sub-criterion 5.2	What the P.O. does to develop and provide services and products oriented to the citizen/customer.
Sub-criterion 5.3	What the P.O. does to develop innovative processes with the citizens' participation.
6th Criterion: Citizens-Oriented rEsults	It assesses the results of the P.O. in relation to the satisfaction of the external and internal customers. It includes 2 sub-criteria.
Sub-criterion 6.1	Results of the citizens'/customers' satisfaction surveys.
Sub-criterion 6.2	Indicators regarding evaluations for citizens/customers.
7th Criterion: Human Resources-oriented Results	It assesses the results that the P.O. achieves in relation to the satisfaction of its human resources. It includes through 2 sub-criteria.
Sub-criterion 7.1	Results of human resources' satisfaction survey.
Sub-criterion 7.2	Indicators of effectiveness of human resources.
8th Criterion: Society-Oriented Results	It assesses what the P.O. achieves for the satisfaction of the needs and expectations of society for topics like the quality of life, the maintenance of global resources, etc. It includes 2 sub-criteria.
Sub-criterion 8.1	What results has the P.O. achieved to address the needs of society in relation to the results of social surveys, as the involved citizens perceive them.
Sub-criterion 8.2	What results has the P.O. achieved to meet the society's needs in relation to indicators of social performance established by the P.O.
9th Criterion: Key Performance Results	It assesses what the P.O. achieves in relation to its constitutional mandate and its defined objectives, as well as in relation to the satisfaction of the needs and expectations of all parties that have a financial interest or participate in the P.O. It includes 2 sub-criteria.
Sub-criterion 9.1	External results. Output- results in relation to the objectives.
Sub-criterion 9.2	Internal results.

Source: (Efkarpidis, 2016).

INTERCONNECTED FUNCTIONS IN THE CONTEXT OF THE CAF STANDARD

The holistic approach of the CAF does not only suggest that one Public Organization's functions are thoroughly assessed but also that all integral elements of the organization are interdependent. The following remarks can be made:

- There is a cause-effect relationship between the left part (conditions-causes) and the right part (results- consequences) of the standard (Figure 2).
- There is a holistic relationship among causes (conditions).

The verification of the interconnection between cause-effect is of fundamental importance for the self-assessment, in the context of which the organization must always check the consistency between certain result or a series of similar results and the evidence arisen from the relevant criteria and sub-criteria regarding conditions. This consistency is sometimes difficult to verify because, due to the holistic character of the organization, the different causes (conditions) interact between each other during the delivery of results. Since the integrity of results is defined largely by the type and intensity of the relationships between conditions, these relationships must be investigated during the assessment. In fact, the intensity of these relationships differs among different organizations and their nature defines largely the quality of the organization.

Aparently the relationships are not limited to the level of criteria. Quite often substantial interactions- relationships exist at the level of sub-criteria.

COMMON EUROPEAN VALUES OF THE PUBLIC SECTOR

The CAF is designed specifically for the Public Sector and this is the differentiating point from the EFQM standard.

Quality in the Public Sector present some unique features compared to the Private Sector, taking into account the basic conditions of the European socio-political and administrative culture (EIPA, 2019).

These conditions are the legitimacy (democratic and parliamentary) and the state of justice and ethics, which are based on common values and principles, like transparency, accountability, participation, diversity, equality, social justice, solidarity, collaboration and the relationships with the stakeholders (EIPA, 2019). All the above constitute elements to be taken into account during the assessment.

Although the CAF focuses mainly on the assessment of the performance of the administration and on the identification of the organizational causes that make improvement possible, the ultimate goal is to contribute to good governance.

THE IMPORTANCE OF EVIDENCE AND MEASUREMENTS OF THE CAF

The self-assessment and the improvement of the Public Organizations become difficult without reliable information from their different functions. The CAF supports Public Organizations in the collection and use of information, yet quite often this information is not available during the first self-assessment. For this reason, the CAF is often seen as measurement that starts from scratch, indicating the important areas for the initiation of the measurement. As long as the Administration is under a process of continuous improvement, information will be increasingly collected and managed in a systemic and gradual manner both in the internal and external environment (Dimitriou and Archontas, 2015).

COMMON ADMINISTRATIVE LANGUAGE AND GLOSSARY OF THE CAF

Many Public Organizations are facing difficulties in understanding Management terminology. The CAF creates a common language allowing the organization's personnel and leadership to discuss about organizational topics in a constructive way. This simple and understandable language by all public employees promotes the dialogue and the bench learning among Public Administrations at European level (Dimitriou and Archontas, 2015).

THE ROLE OF THE ASSESSMENT SYSTEM IN THE CAF

Although the identification of the strengths, the areas for improvements and the relevant improvement actions constitute the most important results of the self-assessment, the CAF scoring system plays an equal special role (Dimitriou and Archontas, 2015).

The scoring of each criterion and sub-criterion of the CAF standard has 4 main objectives:

- To provide an indication for the direction that the Public Organization shall follow as regards improvement actions,
- To measure the improvement of the Public Organization,
- To identify successful practices, as these are determined by the high scores for the conditions and the results &
- To assist in finding the appropriate stakeholders from whom the Public Organization can learn.

SUPPORT IN THE USE OF THE CAF

In 2001 with decision of the responsible General Managers for the Public Administration, a network of national representatives for the CAF was established, as well as the CAF Resource Center, as previously mentioned. This network is responsible at European level for the development and the monitoring of the standard. In addition, it studies new tools and strategies for the promotion of the CAF. CAF Resource Center operates in EIPA in Maastricht, Netherlands and is responsible for the coordination of the network. In addition, it manages the CAF webpage, which is the access point to all CAF-related information and other TQM topics.

In the countries-members of European Union the national representatives take the right initiatives to encouragne and support the use of the standard in their countries. The activities of the Center cover a broad spectrum, ranging from the creation of national centers of data management to the construction of specialized web portals and from national or regional projects or programs to national awards or quality conferences based on the CAF standard (Dimitriou and Archontas, 2015).

THE PROCESS OF EXTERNAL FEEDBACK

In order for the Public Organizations to implement the CAF successfully, there is a formal process to provide feedback from the external environment on the overall quality management with the CAF use. This external feedback process, implemented on a voluntary basis, aims at supporting even more the CAF users on their way towards quality, making their efforts visible within and outside the organization. This feedback process relates to the self-assessment process, as well as to the broader vision of the organizations to achieve excellence over time.

The external feedback process aims at achieving the following objectives:
- To support the quality of the CAF implementation and the impact on the organization,
- To investigate whether the organization adopts the TQM principles, as a consequence of the CAF implementation,
- To support and empower the feeling of enthusiasm with continuous improvement inside the organization,
- To promote the assessment and the bench learning from similar organizations,

- To reward the organizations that have started their course towards continuous improvement for achieving excellence in an effective manner, without criticizing their current quality level &
- To enable the participation of the CAF users at the level of excellence of the EFQM model

The process of the external feedback is based on the following 3 pillars:

- Pillar 1: Self-assessment process,
- Pillar 2: Improvement actions process &
- Pillar 3: Maturity of the organization towards TQM

The organizations that have used the CAF effectively may assume the title of "Effective CAF user" given for a duration of 2 years. The process of external feedback and the previous title are at the discretion of countries-members, which create the practical details having as basis a commonly agreed frame but at their own pace. The organizations that wish to submit an application for the title above have to be informed in advance if this possibility exists in their countries (Dimitriou and Archontas, 2015).

ADVANTAGES OF THE CAF STANDARD

The CAF has the following advantages (Michalopoulos, Polykratis and Dimitriou, 2017):

1. It constitutes a first attempt to manage the diversity of the administrative systems of the countries-members of the European Union, setting common criteria and a single assessment method, so that its conclusions be comparable, commonly accepted and utilizable and common policies be designed if and when conditions allow for it.

2. It allows the development of contacts, communication and cooperation among the agencies of the Public Administration of the countries-members of the European Union, as well as the exchange of experiences for topics of administrative organization and function.
3. It creates the preconditions for the implementation of a broader plan to establish the European Quality Award in the Public Administration.
4. It significantly contributes to the introduction of the philosophy and the concepts of TQM and of Public Management into the Public Organizations.
5. It enforces the participation of the staff of one Public Organization in the process of the assessment of its function, since in principle it is about a self-assessment method.
6. It constitutes a holistic study of the structure and function of one Public Organization at one specific point of time. The self-assessment process is based on real facts and justified conclusions for each aspect under evaluation and it can be carried out by the employees of the Public Organization themselves, without assistance from external partners.
7. Its implementation is a continuous process, since the conclusions of one assessment lead to the implementation of a plan with actions for the improvement of the administrative function, which after their implementation, are re-assessed based on the CAF again.
8. The CAF does not concern the assessment of the public policies that one Public Organization applies, but its administrative function.
9. The CAF is linked in no way with the performance assessment of the personnel of the Public Organization at any hierarchical level of responsibility.
10. The CAF may be implemented either to the whole Organization either to individual units, yet always in an integrated way, as single system and not in a fragmented way with the selective implementation of some criteria and sub-criteria.

CONCLUSION

Concluding on the above observations about the CAF, its implementation is suggested for the Public Organizations, so that they can use a tool for the improvement of their administrative capacity, which belongs to them and they do not necessarily need to refer to external sources for the implementation of some similar integrated methodology.

REFERENCES

Deming Cycle (PDCA). (2000). In: Swamidass P.M. (eds) *Encyclopedia of Production and Manufacturing Management.* Springer, Boston, MA.

Dimitriou, I. and Archontas, N. (2015). *The Common Assessment Framework (CAF) Improving the public organisations through self-assessment, CAF 2013.* Athens: Ministry of internal affairs and administrative reconstruction division of administrative reform and electronic governance general directorate of reform policy and electronic governance directorate of organizational reforms.

Efkarpidis, A. (2016). The implementation of Common Assessment Framework in the assessment of the administrative function and performance of nursery service: the case of one General Hospital of island area. *Hellenic Magazine of Nursery Science,* 9(3), pp. 34-43.

EIPA. (2019). *European CAF Resource Centre - EIPA.* [online] Available at: https://www.eipa.eu/portfolio/european-caf-resource-centre/ [Accessed 21 Jul. 2019].

Engel, C. (2002). Common Assessment Framework: the state of affairs. *Eipascope,* pp.35-9.

Michalopoulos, N., Polykratis, D. and Dimitriou, I. (2017). *Common assessment implementation guide.* 5th ed. Athens: Ministry of internal affairs and administrative reconstruction division of administrative reform and electronic governance general directorate of reform policy and electronic governance directorate of organizational reforms.

Staes, P., Thijs, N., Stoffels, A. and Geldof, S. (2011). *Five Years of CAF 2006 : From Adolescence to Maturity – What Next ?*. p.160.

Tomazevic, N., Seljak, J. and Aristovnik, A. (2014). The impact of CAF enablers on job satisfaction: the case of the Slovenian law enforcement agency. *Total Qual Manag Bus Excell,* 25, pp.1336–51.

BIOGRAPHICAL SKETCHES

Stella Korouli

Affiliation:
Roche Products Limited

Education:
- Post-graduate studies in Design & Management of Health Services- Medical School of Athens University
- Post-graduate studies in Medicinal Chemistry- Design & Synthesis of agents with potential anticancer properties- Pharmacy School of Athens University
- Bachelor in Pharmacy- Pharmacy School of Athens University

Business Address: Roche Products Limited
6 Falcon Way
Shire Park
Welwyn Garden City
AL7 1TW
United Kingdom

Research and Professional Experience:
- Drug Safety
- Patient Safety
- Pharmacovigilance

- Risk Management Plans
- Safety Communications
- Medical Information
- Total Quality Management
- Common Assessment Framework
- Design & Synthesis of agents with potential anticancer properties

Professional Appointments:
- October 2019- present: Patient Safety Manager UK DS Center (International Assignment), Roche Products Limited
- July 2019- September 2019: Drug Safety Manager UK DS Center (International Assignment), Roche Products Limited
- 2016- June 2019: Drug Safety Manager/Local Safety Responsible, Roche (Hellas) SA
- 2015-2016: Head of Drug Safety & Medical Information, Roche (Hellas) SA
- 2011-2014: Drug Safety & Medical Information Manager, Roche (Hellas) SA
- 2010: Drug Safety Manager, Roche (Hellas) SA
- 2008-2010: Drug Safety Associate, Roche (Hellas) SA
- 2006-2008: Clinical Trials Application Officer, Roche (Hellas) SA

Honors:
Awarded Top Performers Award on year 2013 in Roche (Hellas) SA for continuous outstanding performance

Vasiliki Kapaki

Affiliation:
School of Social and Political Sciences, University of Peloponnese, Corinth, Greece

Education:
- Postdoctoral Research Fellow in Health Economics, University of Peloponnese, Corinth, Greece
- Doctor of Philosophy – PhD in Health Policy - Quality of HealthCare Services and Patient Safety, University of Peloponnese, Corinth Greece
- Master of Science (MSc) in Health Economics and Management, University of Piraeus, Greece
- Bachelor in Social Policy, Panteion University, Athens, Greece

Business Address:
44-46 Kriton street, 117 44, Athens, Greece

Research and Professional Experience:
- Consulting Services in Health Policy, Health Economics, Pharmacoeconomics, Drug Evaluation and Health Technology Assessment
- Quality of Healthcare Services
- Total Quality Management
- Patient Safety
- Drug Safety
- Risk Management in Healthcare Organizations (adverse events, medical errors and near misses management)

Professional Appointments:
- Nov. 2018- present: Scientific Member of the Greek Health Technology Assessment Committee
- 2016- present: Postdoctoral Research Fellow in Health Economics, University of Peloponnese, Corinth, Greece
- 2015-Sep.2018: External Health Policy Consultant, Institute of Health Policy, Athens, Greece
- 2015-present: Teaching and Research Staff in Postgraduate programmes in University of Peloponnese, Corinth, Greece and in

Medical School of National and Kapodistrian University of Athens, Greece
- 2014-2015: Research Fellow in Health Policy, University of Peloponnese, Corinth, Greece
- 2010-2013: Research Fellow in Health Policy and Health Economics, National School of Public Health, Athens, Greece

Publications from the Last 3 Years:
- Souliotis K, Golna C, Kotsopoulos N, Kapaki V, Dalucas C. (2018). *Meningitis B vaccination: knowledge and attitudes of pediatricians and parents in Greece.* Heliyon;11;4(11):e00902.
- Kapaki, V. (2018). The anatomy of medication errors. In Dr. Stanislaw Stawicki (Ed.), *Vignettes in Patient Safety* - Volume 4. ISBN 978-953-51-6916-1.
- Kapaki, V. & Souliotis, K. (2018). Defining adverse events and determinants of medical errors in healthcare. In Dr. Stanislaw Stawicki (Ed.), *Vignettes in Patient Safety* - Volume 3. ISBN 978-953-51-6155-4.
- Kapaki, V. & Souliotis, K. (2017). Psychometric properties of the Hospital Survey on Patient Safety Culture (HSOPSC): Findings from Greece. In M.S. Firstenberg and S.P. Stawicki (Ed.), *Vignettes in Patient Safety* - Volume 2. ISBN 978-953-51-5757-1.
- Kapaki, V. & Souliotis, K. (2017). Patient Safety and Medical Errors: Building Safer Healthcare Systems for Better Care. In M. Riga (Ed.), *Impact of Medical Errors and Malpractice on Health Economics, Quality, and Patient Safety* (pp. 61-90). Hershey, PA: IGI Global. doi:10.4018/978-1-5225-2337-6.ch003.
- Kapaki, V. & Souliotis, K. (2017). Patient Safety Culture in Greece: Narrowing the Gap between the Pronciples of Patient Safety Culture and Current Clinical Practice. In E.Williams (Ed.), *Patient Safety and Management: Perspectives, Principles and Emerging Issues* (pp. 87 -117). Nova Science Publisher Inc.

Adamantia Englezopoulou

Affiliation:
- Member of EU Expert Group on Patient Safety and Quality of Care http://ec.europa.eu/health/patient_safety/events/index_en.htm
- Vice-President of the National Committee on Rare and Complicated Diseases
- Greek National Accreditation Council Expert (EN ISO 15224:2012)
- Member of a Peripheral Expert Group on Healthcare Associated Infections and Antimicrobial Resistance

Education:
- Panteion University-Graduate School of Public Administration Greek
- National School of Public Health-postgraduate student on "Health Management"

- Universita Degli Studi Dell' Aquila-Italy-postgraduate student on Master Level II Epidemiology of Health Services, Health Effects and Quality Management of Health Care Services (Epidemiologia Valutativa, Impatto Sanitario e Qualita Delle Aziende Sanitarie)
- PhD candidate in Quality and Patient Safety in Operating Theatre

Business Address:
Saint Thomas St 17 – 115 27 Athens, Greece

Research and Professional Experience:

- Member of an Expert Group:
  - Action Plan for prevention and control of Infection Controls and Microbial Resistance
  - Strategic and Business Plan of Public Hospital
  - Action Plan for Organization of Operating Theatre

- Action Plan for Risk Management of Public Hospital
- Instructor of National Centre for Public Administration and Local Government (National Strategic Agent for the development of the Human Resources of the Public Administration and Local Government)-*Certification No 767/29.01.2014.*
  - Common Assessment Framework
  - Total Quality Management
  - Patient Safety
  - Quality Improvement in Healthcare-Quality Indicators
  - Accreditation of Healthcare Services
- Instructor at Seminars titled:
  - Hospital Risk Management
  - Human Resources Management
  - Quality Management Systems
  - Organization and Management of Healthcare Services
  - Communication and Team Working in Operating Theatre
  - BalancedScoreCard, etc.

Professional Appointments:
- 2019-present: Deputy Manager of General Hospital of Athens "LAIKO".
- 2012-2019: Head of Quality Control, Research and Continuing Education Department of General Hospital of Athens "Sismanoglio-Amalia Flemig".
- 2014-2017: Head of General Secretary Department of General Hospital of Athens "Sismanoglio-Amalia Flemig".
- 2005-2012: Head of Secretary of Outpatient and Emergency Department of General Hospital of Athens "Sismanoglio-Amalia Flemig".
- 2004-2011: Secretary of Administrative Council of General Hospital of Athens "Sismanoglio-Amalia Flemig".
- 2002-2004: Employee of Human Resources Department of General Hospital of Athens "Sismanoglio-Amalia Flemig".

- 1995-2002: Employee of Supplies/Resources Department of General Hospital of Athens "Sismanoglio-Amalia Flemig".
- 1991-1995: Secretary of Technical Department of General Hospital of Athens "Sismanoglio-Amalia Flemig".
- 1985-1991: Secretary of Administrative Council of General Hospital of Athens "Sismanoglio-Amalia Flemig".
- 1983-1985: Employee of General Secretary Department of General Hospital of Athens "Sismanoglio-Amalia Flemig".

Honors:
- Health and Safety Awards 2019-Bronze "Preparedness for a Catastrophic Emergencies".
- Healthcare Business Awards 2018-Silver "Quality System in Emergency Department of Public Hospital".

Publications from the Last 3 Years:
1. Koutalas, E, Englezopoulou, A, Lilis, D, Begkos, K, Demitriadis, G, Apistolas, S, Petrpopoulou, S., Arkoumani, T., Michalakoukos, I., Implementation of the Common Assessment Framework (CAF) as a quality management instrument in a hospital outpatients' department, *Archives of Hellenic Medicine 2019*, 36(6):835–839
2. Englezopoulou, A, Kechagia, M, Chatzikiriakou, R, Kanellopoulou, M, Valenti, M and Masedu, F, Pre Analytical Errors as Quality Indicators in Clinical Laboratory, *Austin J Public Health Epidemiol* - Volume 3 Issue 5 – 2016.
3. Michaelidis, St., K. Tsakanika, Ad. Englezopoulou, C. Paraskevopoulos, A. Petoumenou, E. Kourtelelessi, G. Goulas, "The role of the combined assessment of the Bronchoalveolar Lavage (BAL) and radiological profile in the diagnosis of Chronic Eosinophilic Pneumonia (CEP)", *European Respiratory Society Annual Congress* 2013.
4. Apostolakis, I., Ad. Englezopoulou, *Web 2.0 application in medical and nursing education*, 2012, 101(6) 432-447.

In: Investigating Patient Safety
Editor: Gloria Hale
ISBN: 978-1-53617-344-4
© 2020 Nova Science Publishers, Inc.

Chapter 4

PATIENT SAFETY WITHOUT PATIENT ADVOCACY IS IMPROBABLE, AS THEY ARE SYNONYMOUS: IS THERE A THEORY-PRACTICE-ETHICS GAP?

Manfred Mortell[*], RN, PhD
Department of Nursing, Faculty of Medicine and Health Sciences, University Malaysia Sarawak, Sarawak, Malaysia

ABSTRACT

The aim of a culture of safety in healthcare is to reduce and/or eliminate the risk of harm to patients. However, despite a universal stance towards patient safety, since the Institute of Medicine's landmark report of 2000, *"To Err is Human, building a safer health system"* there remains a disturbing escalation in the healthcare errors among hospitalized patients. This underscores trepidations about healthcare professionals and providers' aptitude as effective and caring patient advocates to provide high quality, safe care. In the context of these healthcare mistakes, the *"Theory-Practice gap"* is often cited as an offending perpetrator. Within this exemplar, there is often a disparity between theoretical knowledge and its

---

[*] Corresponding Author's Email: manny@unimas.my.

application in practice. Evidence relating to the non-integration of theory and practice makes the assumption, that educational dynamics may affect learning and practice outcomes and hence, the *"Gap"*. Whatever you call them, healthcare mistakes, medical errors, faults, or miscalculations. This exemplar, acknowledges that healthcare professionals and providers are provided with theoretical knowledge and prepared with skills to practice competently and safely. Yet, these same healthcare professionals and providers continue to be noncompliant with the recommended evidence-based practices which creates an ethical dilemma. Therefore, to bridge the gap between theory and practice, a *"Theory-Practice-Ethics gap"* must be considered when appraising the unacceptable outcomes in healthcare practices, and the failure of healthcare professionals and providers to fulfil their moral duty of care, as patient advocates.

One of the defining characteristics of a patient advocate is to ensure patient safety. By convention, patient advocacy is an integral philosophy in healthcare, and an obligation which is expected to be fulfilled by healthcare professionals and providers in the course of discharging their duties. *Primum non nocere 'above all, do no harm'* is a fundamental concept within the healthcare model. However, there is evidence of a failure to implement of this moral concept which relates to a patient's safety and the advocacy role expected from healthcare professionals. Healthcare professionals declare that this is because of the ambiguity associated with the comprehension of the advocacy concept in relation to the safety role. In addition to the challenge of role acceptance within a patient safety forum as a misunderstood and unappreciated responsibility. The analytical exploration of patient advocacy related to patient safety and the concept of a *"Theory-Practice-Ethics gap"* will be presented within this chapter, to reinforce the importance of their synonymous relationship for trustworthy healthcare practices. Healthcare professionals and providers need to be mindful of the importance of patient advocacy and the utilization of a safety science which leads to a higher quality of safe patient care.

Keywords: advocate, ethics, medical error, quality, safety, theory-practice-gap

Key Points

Quality Patient Care

The Institute of Medicine defines quality patient care as *"the degree to which healthcare services for individuals and populations increase the likelihood of desired health outcomes and are consistent with current professional knowledge."*

A Culture of Safety

Is the product of individual and group values, attitudes, perceptions, competencies, and patterns of behaviours that determine the commitment to, and the style and proficiency of, an organization's health and safety management!

Patient Safety

Is the prevention of errors and adverse effects to patients associated with health care!

Advocacy

The American Nurses Association deems that advocacy is a pillar of nursing. Nurses instinctively support and protect their patients, in their workplaces, and in the community.

Healthcare Ethics

Autonomy, beneficence, non-maleficence, justice are the fundamental healthcare principles which bioethicists often denote when evaluating the ethical issues related to healthcare procedures and health care decisions.

Theory-Practice-Ethics Gap

A process of noncompliance to ethical evidence based practices despite having the relevant knowledge.

INTRODUCTION

The basis for this chapter is to provoke nurses and other healthcare professionals and providers to consider a dilemma which affects patient care and safety. A dilemma in the literature which has been cited as a *"Theory-Practice-Ethics gap"* (Mortell et al., 2013). Patient safety and high quality of care are essential aspects of all healthcare practices. When people are admitted to hospital, they expect to have their illness, disorder or disease treated effectively, and receive safe, high quality care during the process. They do not expect to be put at risk or be harmed, since the principal goal of healthcare is to maximize care, safety and wellbeing, and so optimize the quality of people's lives (*Leape, 2015;* Wilson et al., 2009).

Nursing has been termed the caring profession, and as such, a nurse as a healthcare professional and provider is often required to perform multidimensional roles. One of those roles is as a patient advocate, a responsibility which is often challenging due to composite interactions between nurses, patients, professional colleagues, and the community (Mortell et al., 2017). Nevertheless, despite the demands of the role, nursing has embraced advocacy as a professional paradigm. Advocacy has numerous meanings and conventions, but in nursing it is generally depicted as representing another, whilst endeavouring to protect the health, safety, and the rights of the patient (Mathews, 2012; American Nurses Association, 2010). The nurse as a patient advocate therefore, plays a key role to keep patients safe throughout their encounters within the health care systems. As a vocation, nursing is a demanding undertaking, and the added responsibility of patient advocacy is particularly strenuous for nurses given the intricacy of their duties in the healthcare setting. In addition to the procedural care responsibilities which maybe complex, nurses also have the added responsibility for patient safety, which is often subject to ethical and moral challenges (Monterosso et al., 2005). Therefore, nurses have an ethical obligation to keep the patient safe to prevent harm (Joint Commission International, 2010; Institute of Medicine, 2000).

The word ethics has Greek origins; Ta Ethika: into good and evil; Ethos: personal character. A code of ethics defines basic principles to determine what constitutes "*right*" behaviour, united with a moral duty and obligation. Ethics are moral values and behaviours that express ideals for other human beings, comprising of commitments to remove harm and/or promote benefit (Twomey, 2010). The fundamental principles for patient safety management, "P*rimum non nocere*" (first do no harm) and "*In dubio abstine*" (in case of doubt, do not intervene) go back to ancient times. Historically, Hippocrates, a Greek physician born circa 460 BC is acknowledged as the father of medicine and was concerned with alleviating human suffering whilst pledging ethical values and moral conduct. He conceived the Hippocratic Oath to remind physicians to practice medicine ethically, ensure safe and effective care and never do any harm.

In similarity, the nursing profession and hence nurses abide by an equivalent oath, referred to as the Nightingale pledge. This pledge reminds nurses of their obligations to the patient, as perceived by Florence Nightingale more than 150 years ago. Her expressed concern was that the greatest threat to patient safety were the "*frailties of the human condition, complacent attitudes and unconscious behaviours*" (Reid, 2011). These are patient safety practice issues and concerns which remain applicable in today's healthcare climate.

Therefore, patient safety and high quality of care are and remain essential aspects of all healthcare practices, and whilst the medical profession focuses on the clinical, scientific and ethical competence aimed at curing and healing those people who are unwell. The Nursing profession concentrates on the moral and ethical work of the health experience for a human-being by caring for them physically, emotionally, and spiritually. Both the Hippocratic Oath and the Nightingale pledge for all intents and purposes promote patient advocacy and safety.

A CULTURE OF SAFETY IN HEALTHCARE

Safety is a fundamental facet of healthcare and an organizational ethos for the patient's wellbeing acknowledges strategies such as leadership; teamwork; evidence based practice; communication; education; just culture;

and patient centeredness for successful outcomes (Sammer, 2010). However, the time-honoured literature cautioned that despite the placement of well-defined safety strategies, the incidence of healthcare errors may not decrease due to the high incidence of violations by healthcare professionals and providers which create patient safety issues (O'Shea (1999). This caveat appears to be validated by the Institute of Medicine's report of 2000, that despite the application of organizational safety strategies, healthcare errors continue to occur frequently which compromises patient care and safety (Makary, & Daniel, 2016; Leape 2015; Institute of Medicine, 2006). These enduring healthcare errors, could be explained by the healthcare professionals and provider's behavioural attitudes toward the recommended safe practice organizational strategies, non-compliance, or deliberate violations regarding administrative guidelines (Dean et al. 2008; Lachman, 2007).

In the context of healthcare errors, the *"Theory-Practice gap"* is often cited by academics as the offending educational perpetrator due to outdated information (Mahmoud, 2014). Within this *"Theory-Practice"* paradigm there is often a gap between theoretical knowledge and its application in practice, which will affect learning and practice outcomes (Saifan et al., 2015). Yet, education programs which were introduced following the Institute of Medicine report (2000) to improve healthcare professionals and provider's knowledge, and practices to decrease healthcare errors, have demonstrated negligible improvement with continuing practice violations (Makary, & Daniel, 2016; Schneider, 2006). Therefore, from a perspective of healthcare errors, as organizations adopt more complex strategies to improve patient safety, success of these strategies will still depend on professional responsibility, accountability, and practice ethics. Hence, to bridge the gap between *"Theory and Prac*tice*"* an additional factor called *"Ethics"* is required, and must be considered (Mortell, 2009).

The nursing literature also implies a crisis of ethics where *"Theory and Prac*tice*"* integrate, and that we as healthcare professionals and providers are failing to full fill our duty as patient advocates (Mortell et al., 2017; Mortell, 2017; 2012). Endeavours must therefore be made to encourage ethical practices and have healthcare professionals and providers reflect on their moral duty, as advocates to provide safe, quality patient care. Only by creating a culture of ethical care as patient advocates can we hope to decrease the '*Theory-Practice-Ethics gap*' and preserve patient safety.

PERCEPTIONS OF PATIENT ADVOCACY

Despite the recurring use of the term "*advocacy*" in the health sciences literature, and its presence in academic curricula, there remains a contrasting opinion about advocacy and the role for nurses. The patient advocate is often perceived as that of being the patient "*protector*" *or* "*defender*", which is endorsed by numerous authors (Kupperschmidt, 2014; American Nurses Association, 2010). Nurses consider themselves foremost as the "*protectors*" of vulnerable patients (White et al., 2014). These nurses as "*protectors*" often have patient safety concerns related to the unnecessary, insensitive and often inhumane care, which do not advocate for the patient (Kupperschmidt, 2014; Jowers-Ware et al., 2011). A fundamental prerequisite that obligates nurses to act as an advocate is patient vulnerability (White et al., 2014).

Traditionally, the epitome of a nurse was defined as a champion of the sick, a healer, a counsellor and health educator. Nursing has been defined as "*the protection, promotion, and optimization of health and abilities, prevention of illness and injury, alleviation of suffering through the diagnosis and treatment of the human response, and advocacy in the care of individuals, families, communities and popula*tions" (American Nursing Association, 2003, p. 6). Curtin (1983) humorously declared, that the nurse as a patient advocate is "*a combination lawyer-theologian-psychologist-family counsellor and dragon slayer wrapped in a white uniform*" (p. 154). Advocacy has also been depicted as an "*ethical ideal*" (Davis et al. 2003) with a fundamental criterion that requires nurses to act as a patron for the vulnerable patient, whether in terms of individual vulnerability due to illness or injury or as a consequence of intrinsic risks which may be encountered within the healthcare system (Bu et al., 2006). Nurses therefore perform a fundamental role as a patient advocate to ensure that the treatment and care offered is apt and safe (Selanders & Crane, 2012). However, the obstacles that challenge nurses as patient advocates are often problematic and well documented in the literature (Davoodvand, Abbaszadeh & Ahmadi, 2016; Black, 2011; Sack, 2010). Despite the acknowledged importance of the advocacy role, it has also been conceded that the role may have both positive and negative consequences. While it provides patient benefits, such as quality care and enhanced safety, it exposes the patient advocate to various potential challenges. This is especially true when the nurse advocate's duty of care requires intervention interacts with power structures within the multidisciplinary healthcare team and the employing organisation (Mortell et al., 2017).

The obvious benefits of patient advocacy include dependable, safe patient care, enhanced liaison with the patient and family and greater cooperation with allied multi-disciplinary healthcare professionals (Kupperschmidt, 2014; Thacker, 2008). In addition to empowerment of the patient, protection of their rights and values, and ensuring that patient autonomy is preserved (Bu et al. 2006). Nurse researchers such as Vaartio & Leino-Kilpi, (2004) reported that advocacy interventions by nurses provided unquestionable positive health outcomes, especially in the context of vulnerable, at risk age populations, such as infants and the elderly. For nurses the identified advocacy benefits included that society regarded nurses as dependable, honest, and reliable, which has enhanced the communal image and professional status of nurses and the nursing profession (Bu et al., 2006).

However, there were also various detriments and aftermaths from nurse colleagues, other healthcare professionals and providers and the employing organisation for nurses choosing to act as patient advocates (Mortell et al., 2017; Mallik, 1997a, 1997b, 1997c). Nurses as patient advocates have been labelled as trouble makers by colleagues, accused of insubordination, and have suffered loss of self-esteem, friends, reputation, and career advancement (Mortell et al., 2017; Bu et al., 2006; Vaartio & Leino-Kilpi, 2004). The logic for these negative outcomes was that a nurse's advocacy actions could threaten the nurse-doctor relationship, especially if their actions countered the physician's patient care decisions. In addition to identified advocacy issues which contradicted organizational ideals. Healthcare organisations normally require employees to adhere to administrative policies and procedures. Nurses that attempted to fulfil their ethical obligation as a patient advocate could find their actions challenging, demoralizing and intimidating. In such cases, the nurse is often subjected to the forfeiture of their professional reputation, loss of their self-esteem, the absence of career promotion, or employment dismissal, with subsequent ostracism by co-workers and friends (Mortell et al., 2017; Mallik, 1997a, 1997b, 1997c).

Regardless of the perceptions of advocacy, the significance of advocacy is an undeniable prerequisite to achieving the goal of effective quality patient care and to ensure that patients are safe when they require healthcare. Consistent with one of the most frequently cited views concerning advocacy, Vaartio & Leino-Kilpi (2004) stated that the advocacy must be appreciated in terms of quality health and care, which includes protecting patients from harm (p. 704).

CONSIDER A *"THEORY - PRACTICE - ETHICS GAP"*

A fundamental element essential for patient care and safety which is not emphasized enough in nursing or healthcare is *"ethics"*. This is a moral obligation as a healthcare professional and provider to the patients and their families to ensure that they receive safe, quality care. Although numerous studies have discussed patient advocacy in nursing, and a *"Theory-Practice gap"*, this chapter discloses concerns that relate to patient safety, non-compliance amongst healthcare professionals and providers as patient advocates, and the possibility of a *"Theory-Practice-Ethics gap"*.

The following two case studies will provide the reader with an opportunity to reflect on their own clinical practices and serve as prudent reminders that everything we do as healthcare professionals and providers has potential ramifications for the patient. In addition to the reflecting on the reality that all healthcare professionals and providers are patient advocates and that all patients regardless of their religion, race, culture, age or gender are entitled to trustworthy, safe, quality care.

Case Study 1

A 46-year-old male was referred from a cardiology clinic to a cardiac surgical clinic with severe refractory angina pectoris with suspected coronary artery disease. Successive investigations confirmed triple vessel coronary artery disease, which would require open chest surgery and coronary artery bypass grafts. The obstructive pathophysiology involved the left anterior descending artery 95%; Left circumflex artery 100%, and right coronary artery 90%. The unstable angina despite maximal medical management had become progressively worse over a period of 6 months. The patient's 12 lead electrocardiograph, demonstrated widespread non ST segment elevation myocardial ischemia.

On clinical examination, he was anxious, had a pulse rate of 110 beats per minute; a systemic blood pressure 130/80 mmHg; Shortness of breath with a respiratory rate of 28 breaths per minute; a SpO2 of 92% on room air. Audible crackles on auscultation throughout bilateral lung fields. Chest x-ray confirmed cardiomegaly, and congestive heart failure. The angina pectoris was stated to be a constant ache, sub-sternal in location, with a degree of left arm numbness and "pain" with a numerical value of 8/10 to 10/10 depending on his physical activity or psychosomatic stresses.

A medical-surgical procedure was recommended to the patient, which was coronary artery bypass grafts as a definitive intervention to circumvent his coronary lesions. On the day of the scheduled surgery, a patient was collected from the cardiology ward and transferred to the operating room. Before commencing the surgery, a final patient verification "TIME OUT", was performed according to hospital policy and the Joint Commission International's patient safety goal, "*Ensure right site; right patient; right procedure–surgery*" (Joint Commission International, 2010). This was done in the presence of the cardiac surgeon, who with astonishment stated that this was the wrong patient and that this patient was not for the scheduled surgical procedure of coronary artery bypass grafts. The surgery was subsequently cancelled and the patient was returned to the recovery unit.

REFLECTING ON THE "NEAR MISS" EVENT

As a healthcare professional and provider identifying a patient correctly prior to any procedure is an established responsibility, whether a procedure is minor or major. Typically, before any medical procedure, the patient's full name and medical record number must be confirmed. Correct identification of a patient prior to any procedure is a standard healthcare practice, which preserves patient safety (Joint Commission International, 2010). There are no routine medical procedures in healthcare, every intervention could place the patient at risk and in harms-way. The patient concerned was incorrectly identified and taken to the operating room for open chest surgery, a major procedure. This surgery would involve opening the chest cavity, commencing cardiopulmonary bypass, harvesting the saphenous vein and radial arteries for the coronary artery bypass grafts and include numerous additional invasive interventions. Employing; the Joint Commission International's patient safety goal number 4; "*Ensure right site; right patient; right procedure–surgery*" (Joint Commission International, 2010) or the equivalent depending on the organization's policy (Emergency Care Research Institute, 2016). All patients must be afforded a safe systematic organizational process to be identified correctly before any procedure. Correct patient identification is a practice which all healthcare professionals and providers, have been informed and instructed on, with subsequent compliance being validated.

This "*Near miss*" event demonstrates that there is a "*theory-practice-ethics gap*". When healthcare professionals and providers are non-compliant within their practice, despite being ratified by their profession and prepared by their employing organization to provide ethical care which has been fortified with the relevant evidence-based theory and practice. The case study focuses on two issues which relate to patient care and safety, the first is an ongoing medical dilemma, which involved correct patient identification. The second, an issue which revealed a potential conflict of professional ethics within a new paradigm called the "*theory-practice-ethics gap*". This paradigm, acknowledges that all healthcare professionals and providers are provided with theoretical knowledge and functional skills to practice competently and safely. Yet, these same healthcare professionals and providers continue to be ethically non-compliant in their clinical practice, which creates an ethical patient safety dilemma.

Case Study 2

A 3-year-old toddler was brought into emergency department of a tertiary hospital by his parents. The father informed the emergency department nursing staff that the toddler had been unwell with a cough and fever for several days. The emergency department nursing staff recorded the following observations. A fever with a core temperature of 38.5°C, rigor like shivering, rapid, shallow breathing, an SpO2 88% on room air, chest retractions, and fatigue. During the ensuing history undertaking by the emergency department physician, when asked about allergy status, the parents stated that the toddler had developed a severe rash and breathing difficulties following the administration of an oral Penicillin suspension on a previous occasion. The Penicillin allergy status of the toddler was documented and flagged in the physician's hand-written and electronic medical records. Succeeding investigations included laboratory tests, such as nasopharyngeal bacterial swabs, blood cultures, and a complete blood count which highlighted a high white cell count of 15,000/mm^3; neutrophils 70%, bands 15%, lymphocytes 15%. An Anterior-Posterior chest x-ray was also recorded.

The toddler was commenced on oxygen therapy which elevated the SpO2 to 94% and was subsequently transferred to the Paediatric High Dependency Unit for specialist care, close monitoring and the commencement of prophylactic antibiotic therapy. On arrival in the Paediatric High Dependency Unit, the toddler's physical examination findings by nursing staff revealed that the toddler was drowsy, had a pulse rate of 138 beats per minute; a systemic blood pressure of 104/63 mmHg; a respiratory rate of 55 breaths per minute with associated shortness of breath, and an SpO2 of 92% on oxygen 40% non-rebreather mask. Pulmonary auscultation revealed wheezing and decreased air entry on the right side of the chest. The chest x-ray verified a right sided middle and lower lobe abnormality and probable pneumonia.

Once the toddler was settled, the Paediatric High Dependency Unit physician prescribed intravenous Amoxicillin as antibiotic prophylaxis until the culture and sensitivity report from laboratory was available to prescribe the specific antibiotic regime. Following the medical prescription of the intravenous Amoxicillin for the toddler, it was then transcribed by the Paediatric High Dependency Unit nurse, and subsequently dispensed from the satellite pharmacy to the Paediatric High Dependency Unit. The intravenous Amoxicillin was then prepared for administration by the primary nurse caring for the toddler. The antibiotic was connected to the toddler's intravenous site and about to be administered intravenously when the parents who were still present at the bedside queried the medication. The father restated to the nurse that their child had a medication allergy to Penicillin. The nurse informed the parents that this medication was not Penicillin, it was Amoxicillin and that they needn't worry as "*she knew what she was doing*". Following the commencement of the intravenous Amoxicillin as prescribed, transcribed, dispensed and administered, the toddler had an anaphylactic reaction and subsequently had a cardiopulmonary arrest.

A paediatric Code Blue was announced over the hospital's public address system, the paediatric Code Blue team arrived within minutes and the toddler was effectively resuscitated. The toddler was then intubated with an oral tracheal tube and was transferred to the paediatric intensive care unit for mechanical ventilation and stabilisation.

Reflecting on the "*Sentinel*" Event

As a healthcare professional and provider, knowledge about pharmaceuticals is a fundamental requirement for all registered nurses in their daily practice (Nursing and Midwifery Council-UK, 2018; World Health Organization, 2010; Australian Commission on Safety and Quality in Health Care, 2013). Before administering any medication to a patient, the nurse must know about the medication administration rights and establish the "*known allergy status*" of the patient (Powrie, 2018). The nurse must also know the rationale for the prescription of the medication, the generic name of the medication, the related medication "*families*", the actions, and potential adverse effects of the medication. These are fundamental medication principles which are established as a nursing practice responsibility. This praxis applies to all medications, whether the medication is oral, nasal, enteral, trans-dermal, sub-cutaneous, intra-muscular, intra-venous, epidural, or intra-thecal.

The benchmark in healthcare practice, before the administration of any medication, is to verify the patient's Full name, Medical Record Number and the documented "*known allergy status*". This practice ensures patient safety and prevents any potential medical error related harm (Joint Commission International, 2010). Nurses, as healthcare professionals, providers and patient advocates are aware that there are no routine medical procedures in healthcare, every medication prescribed and administered could place the patient at risk and in harms-way. Antibiotics such as Penicillin are often used to treat streptococcus infections, as they damage the bacterial cell, inhibit cell wall synthesis, and stop bacterial growth. Penicillin is also a known medication and is interrelated to a "*family*" of antibiotics known as the Beta-lactams, which includes Amoxicillin. Amoxicillin is therefore termed a "*Penicillin-like-antibiotic*". If you are allergic to Penicillin, you may be allergic to other types of Beta-lactams, such as Amoxicillin.

This case study involved a 3-year old toddler who was admitted to the hospital with presumed pneumonia. During the medical examination by the emergency department physician it was noted and documented that the toddler was allergic to Penicillin. An allergy status alert was applied on to the medical records documentation hardcopy and was immediately flagged electronically to the pharmacy department. The toddler was subsequently transferred and admitted to the Paediatric High Dependency Unit by the nursing staff. This was followed by a review of the emergency department medical records documentation and a targeted physical assessment by the Paediatric High Dependency Unit physician. The antibiotic that was subsequently prescribed by the Paediatric High Dependency Unit physician was intravenous Amoxicillin, this medicament was then transcribed by the primary nurse and relayed electronically to the satellite pharmacy. The intravenous Amoxicillin was dispensed by the pharmacist to the Paediatric High Dependency Unit primary nurse caring for the toddler. The intravenous Amoxicillin was administered which resulted in an anaphylactic reaction and cardiopulmonary arrest.

The process of identification and acknowledgement of the toddler's *"known allergy status"* in this case study progressed through four stages of safeguards which should have identified the patient's *"known allergy status"*. These stages included 1. The Paediatric High Dependency Unit physician prescribing the medication, 2. The Paediatric High Dependency Unit nurse transcribing, the medication order, 3. The Pharmacist dispensing the medication, 4. The Paediatric High Dependency Unit nurse administering the medication. However, all of the stages failed to identify the patient's *"known allergy status"* prior to prescribing, transcribing, dispensing and administering the medication, and resulted in the near fatal cardiopulmonary arrest of a 3-year old toddler.

The practice of correct patient identification with medication administration is a standard practice and complies with the recommended Joint Commission International's patient safety goal number 1; *"Identify the correct patient"* (Joint Commission International, 2010). All patients must therefore be correctly identified by their Full name, and Medical Record Number in addition to confirming the *"known allergy status"* and medication administration rights for that drug. This is a standard safety practice which is required from all healthcare professionals and providers who are involved with patient medications.

Irrespective of the contributing issues, whether they are attitudinal behaviours, medical errors, faults, slips, non-compliance problems, questions about ethics. The healthcare professionals and providers who instigated this "*Sentinel event*" neglected to follow the standard policies and practices related to "*known allergy status*" which ensures a patient's safety when receiving a medication. The safeguard failures occurred at multiple levels, which included the Paediatric High Dependency Unit physician; the Paediatric High Dependency Unit nurse, the Pharmacist, and the toddler's parent's concerns about their toddler's allergy status. The failure to acknowledge the "*known allergy status*" could have resulted in fatal consequences associated with the cardiopulmonary arrest for the 3-year old toddler. In a perfect world, healthcare would occur in an exceedingly reliable system where no one is hurt and everyone gets the quality care they need. But, in reality, patients continue to be harmed with the professionals choosing to state that "*we're all human*" and, "*To Err is Human*" (Hinno, Partanen, & Vehviläinen-Julkunen, 2011; James, 2013; Fowler et al., 2008).

This case study focused on two issues which relate to patient safety, the first was an ongoing medical predicament, which involved the identification of a 3-year old toddler's "*known allergy status*". The second, was the issue which exposed a potential conflict of professional ethics within a paradigm called the "*theory-practice-ethics gap*" (Mortell, 2013, 2012). This paradigm, again acknowledges that all healthcare professionals and providers are provided with theoretical knowledge and practical skills to perform competently and safely, yet continue to be ethically non-compliant. Non-compliance to the authorized policy and procedure for clinical practices, such as medication administration creates an ethical dilemma, with potential fatal consequences. It also serves as a cautious and far-sighted reminder that everything we do to or for the patient has potential consequences.

CONCLUSION

In this chapter, viewpoints related to patient safety and quality care were presented and discussed in the context of a "*Theory-Practice-Ethics gap*".

The Institute of Medicine's report '*To Err Is Human: Building a Safer Health System*' stated that patients are frequently placed at risk of morbidity and mortality in the United States of America as a result of medical errors (Institute of Medicine, 2000). European nations also had concerns associated with ongoing medical errors which increase the risk of a patient's morbidity and mortality (Classen, et al., 2011; Hinno, Partanen, & Vehviläinen-Julkunen, 2011). The Institute of Medicine's report (2000) generated questions about patient safety and an obligation for healthcare professionals and providers to deliver high quality, safe healthcare (Institute of Medicine, 2000, 2012). However, despite the transparency that was revealed by the Institute of Medicine's report (2000) and the safety strategies recommended by organizations such as The Joint Commission International; patients continue to experience preventable harm and unacceptable care (Leape, 2015; Dixon-Woods, et al., 2014*)*. Alarmingly, Makary and Daniel, (2016), concurred that the healthcare errors remained prevalent and are considered the third leading cause of death in the United States of America, after heart disease and cancer.

There is no refuting that health care dynamics are complex and involve care processes which include sophisticated technologies and therapeutic interventions. However, with an enlarging world-wide population and an extended human life expectancy, the enduring frequent occurrences of healthcare errors, remain as a patient safety issue and concern.

Historically, the role of a patient advocate was perceived as fundamental for the profession of nursing, as it pledged the patient their rights, and their safety when receiving therapeutic treatment and care. Traditionally, the role of an advocate emphasized the provision of a duty of care; which was also embraced by nurses and the international nursing profession. The obligation for a patient-nurse advocate is therefore regarded as an ethical ideal which is grounded on the notion that nurses provide continuity of care with greater intimacy (Mathews, 2012). The modern-day nursing profession also declares that patient advocacy is a fundamental tenet of nursing practice. Nurses, as health care professionals and providers, practicing within the modern era must therefore question and reason logically why "*ethics*" are important and why they must be integrated with "*Theory and Practice*".

Present-day healthcare integrates the latest evidence based education, which we call '*theory*', and combines this with psycho-motor skills, which we call '*practice*', in order to provide high quality care to achieve the best patient outcomes. However, despite being provided with instruction [theory] and competence assessments [practice] the healthcare errors continue to be commonplace in the healthcare setting (Emergency Care Research Institute, 2016).

The "*Theory-Practice gap*" currently remains a significant topic in nursing, given that it confronts the concept of evidence based practice, which is the foundation of nursing as a profession. Although numerous studies have acknowledged a "*Theory-Practice gap*" this chapter reveals patient safety concerns which relate to healthcare ethics, and a "*Theory-Practice-Ethics gap*". Actions must therefore be taken to promote healthcare ethics and have healthcare professionals and providers reflect on their moral duty, to provide safe, quality patient care. Only by creating a culture of ethical care can we hope to provide safe quality care and decrease the "*theory-practice-ethics gap*". This "*Theory-Practice-Ethics gap*" must be considered when reviewing some of the unacceptable outcomes in health care practice (Mortell, 2009).

REFERENCES

American Nurses Association. (2003). *Code of Ethics for nurses and interpretive statements.* Washington: American Nurses Publishing.

American Nurses Association. (2010). *Scope and standards of practice.* 2nd edn. Silver Spring. [Online]. Available from: www.nursebooks.org. [Accessed: 12 June 2014].

Australian Commission on Safety and Quality in Health Care- Acsqhc (2017). https://www.health.gov.au/internet/budget/publishing. nsf/Content/2017-2018_Health_PBS_sup2/$File/201718_Health_ PBS_4.02_ACSQHC.pdf.

Black, L. (2011). Tragedy into policy: a quantitative study of nurses' attitudes toward patient advocacy activities. *Advanced Journal of*

Nursing. [Online] EBSCO, 111 (6), p. 26-35. Available from: http://www.ebscohost.com. [Accessed: 10 June 2015].

Bu, X. & Jezewski, M. (2006). Developing a midrange theory of patient advocacy through concept analysis. *Journal of Advanced Nursing.* [Online] *EBSCO, 57* (1), p. 101-110. Available from: http://www.ebscohost.com [Accessed: 10 June 2015].

Classen, D, C., Resar, R., Griffin, F., Federico, F., Frankel, T., Kimmel, N., Whittington, J. C., Frankel, A., Seger, A. & James, B. C. (2011). 'Global trigger tool' shows that adverse events in hospitals may be ten times greater than previously measured. *Health Affairs Millwood.*, Apr, *30* (4), 581-9. doi: 10.1377/hlthaff.2011.0190.

Curtin, L. (1983). The nurse as advocate: a cantankerous critique. *Nursing Management.* [Online] *WILEY, 14* (5), p. 9-10. Available from: http://www.onlinelibrary.wiley.com [Accessed: 9 June 2014].

Davis, A. J., Konishi, E. & Tahiro, M. (2003). A pilot study of selected Japanese nurses' ideas on patient advocacy. *Nursing Ethics.* [Online] *WILEY,* (12) *10,* p. 404-413. Available from: http://www.onlinelibrary.wiley.com [Accessed: 10 June 2014].

Davoodvand, S., Abbaszadeh, A. & Ahmadi, F. (2016). Patient advocacy from the clinical nurses' viewpoint: a qualitative study. *J Med Ethics Hist Med., 5* (5), pp. 5 – 7.

Dean, B., et al. (2008). Causes of prescribing errors in hospital inpatients. A prospective study. *Lancet., 359* (9315), pp. 373 – 378.

Dixon-Woods, M., Baker, R., Charles, K., et al. *(2014).* Culture and Behavior in the English National Health Service: Overview of lessons from a large multi-method study. *BMJ Qual Saf, 23, pp.* 106–15. doi: 10.1136/bmjqs-2013-001947.

Emergency Care Research Institute. (2016). *Patient identification errors report*, Emergency Care Research Institute June 2016, Accessed, June 18, 2018.

Fowler, M. (2008). *Guide to the Code of Ethics for Nurses: Interpretation and application.* Silver Spring, MD: American Nurses Association.

Hinno, S., Partanen, P. & Vehviläinen-Julkunen, K. (2011). 'Hospital nurses' work environment, quality of care provided and career plans'.

International Nursing Review, *58*(2), pp. 255–262. http://dx.doi.org/10.1111/j.1466-7657.2010.00851.x.

Institute of Medicine. (2000). *To Err Is Human: Building a Safer Health System*. Washington DC: National Academy Press.

Institute of Medicine. (2006). *Committee on Identifying and Preventing Medication Errors*, DC: The National Academic Press.

Joint Commission International. (2010). *National patient safety goals. The joint Commission*, retrieved from http//www.jointcommission.org. patient safety/national patient safety goals/Nov 3, 2010. Accessed, June 20, 2018.

Jowers Ware, L., Bruckenthal, P., Davis, G. & O'connor-Von, S. (2011). Factors that influence patient advocacy by pain management nurse: results of the American Society for Pain Management nursing survey. *Pain Management Nursing*. [Online] *EBSCO*, *12* (1), pp. 25-32. Available from: http://www.ebscohost.com [Accessed: 6 June 2015].

Kupperschmidt, B. R. (2014). Advocacy : Time to take another look ? *The Oklahoma Nurse*. [Online] *EBSCO*, *59* (1), p. 10. Available from: http://www.ebscohost.com [Accessed: 9th June 2014].

Lachman, V. D. (2007). Patient safety: the ethical imperative. *Medsurg Nurs.*, *16* (6), pp. 401–403.

Leape, L. L. (2015). 'Hospital readmissions following surgery turning complications into treasures', *Journal of the American Medical Association.*, *313* (5) 467–468. http://dx.doi.org/10.1001/jama.2014.18614.3.

Mahmoud, M. H. (2014). 'Practical learning and theory practice gap as perceived by nursing students', *International Journal of Current Research*, *6*, (2) 5083-5093 http://www.journalcra.com, Accessed, May 10, 2018.

Makary, M. & Daniel, M. (2016). 'Medical error-the third leading cause of death in the US', *BMJ*, 353-358. doi: https://doi.org/10.1136/bmj.i2139.

Mallik, M. (1997a). Patient representatives: a new role in patient advocacy. *British Journal of Nursing*. [Online] *WILEY*, *6* (7), p. 108-113. Available from: http://www.onlinelibrary.wiley.com [Accessed: 10 June 2014].

Mallik, M. (1997b). Advocacy in nursing – perceptions of practicing nurses. *Journal of Clinical Nursing*. [Online] *WILEY*, *6* (6), p. 303-313. Available from: http://www.onlinelibrary.wiley.com [Accessed: 10 June 2014].

Mallik, M. (1997c). Advocacy in Nursing – a review of the literature. *Journal of Advanced Nursing* [Online] *WILEY*, 25 (1), p. 130-138. Available from: http://www.onlinelibrary.wiley.com [Accessed: 10 June 2014].

Matthews, J. H. (2012). Role of professional organizations in advocating for the nursing profession. Online *J Issues Nurs.*, *17*(1), pp. 3 - 6.

Monterosso, L., Kristjanson, L., Sly, P., Mulcahy, M., Holland, B. G., Grimwood, S. & White, K. (2005). The role of the neonatal intensive care nurse in decision-making: advocacy, involvement in ethical decisions and communication. *International Journal of Nursing Practice*. [Online] *WILEY*, *11* (3), pp. 108-117. Available from: http://www.onlinelibrary.wiley.com [Accessed: 10 June 2014].

Mortell, M. (2009). A resuscitation dilemma theory-practice-ethics. Is there a theory-practice-ethics gap? *J Saudi Heart Assoc.*, *21* (3) pp. 149-52. doi: 10.1016/j.jsha.2009.06.002. Epub 2009 Aug 5.

Mortell, M. (2012). Hand hygiene compliance: Is there a theory-practice-ethics gap? *British Journal of Nursing*, *21* (17), pp. 5-12. https://doi.org/10.12968/bjon.2012.21.17.1011.

Mortell, M., Balky, H. H., Tannous, E. B. & Jong, M. T. (2013). Physician 'defiance' towards hand hygiene compliance: Is there a theory–practice–ethics gap? *J Saudi Heart Assoc.*, *25*(3), pp. 203–208. doi: 10.1016/j.jsha.2013.04.003.

Mortell, M. (2017). *Patient advocacy among Saudi Arabian adult intensive care nurses: A grounded theory study*. Unpublished doctoral thesis; Kuala Lumpur (Malaysia): Faculty of Nursing and Midwifery, MAHSA University.

Mortell, M.., Abdullah, L. & Ahmad, C. (2017). Barriers deterring patient advocacy in a Saudi Arabian critical care setting. *British Journal of Nursing*, *26* (16), pp. 2-8.

Nursing and Midwifery Council UK. (2018). *Professional standards of practice and behaviour for nurses, midwives and nursing associates.* http://www.nmc.org.uk/standards/code/.

O'shea, E. (1999). Factors contributing to medication errors. *A literature review.*, 199 (8), pp. 496 – 504.

Powrie, K. (2018). Identification and management of drug allergy. *Nursing Standard.*, *33*, pp. 123 – 30. doi: 10.7748/ns2018.e9849.

Reid, J. (2011). Patient safety: a core value in Nursing – so why is achieving so difficult? *Jr of Research in Nursing.*, *16* (3), pp. 209-233.

Sack, K. (2010). *Nurse to stand trial for reporting doctor.* The New York Times, February 7th, 2010, Retrieved from www.nytimes.com/2010/02/07/us/07nurses.html?

Saifan, A. R., Safieh, H. A., Mibes, R. & Shibly, R. (2015). Suggestions to Close the Gap in Nursing Education: Nursing Students' Perspectives. *International Journal of Nursing Didactics*, *5* (10), pp. 380-386. http://dx.doi.org/10.1111/j.1466-7657.2011.00947.x.

Sammer, C. E., Lykens, K., Singh, K. P., Mains, D. A. & Lackan, N. A. (2010). What is a patient safety culture: A review of the literature? *J Nurs Scholarship*, *42*, pp. 156-165, doi: 10.1111/j1547-15069.2009.01330. x.

Schneider, P. J. (2006). Improving the safety of MA using interactive CD-ROM program. *Am J Health Syst. Pharm*, *63*, pp. 59 – 64.

Selanders L. C. & Crane, P. C. (2012). The voice of Florence Nightingale on advocacy. Online *J Issues Nurs.*, *17* (1), pp. 1 – 3.

Thacker, K. S. (2008) Nurses' advocacy behaviours in end of life nursing care. *Nursing Ethics.* [Online] *WILEY*, *15* (8). p. 174-185. Available from: http://www.onlinelibrary.wiley.com [Accessed: 10 June 2014].

Twomey, J. (2010). In *Guide to the code of ethics for nurses.* Interpretation and application in Fowler, Med. Silver Springs MD. ANA.

Vaartio, H. & Leino-Kilpi, H. (2004). Nursing advocacy – a review of the empirical research 1990 – 2003. *International Journal of Nursing Studies.* [Online] *EBSCO 42* (6), p. 705-14. Available from: http://www.ebscohost.com [Accessed: 3 June 2014].

White, K. R., Roczen, M. L., Coyne, P. J. & Wiencek, C. (2014). Acute and critical care nurses' perceptions of palliative competencies: a pilot study. *Journal of Continuing Education in Nursing*. [Online] *EBSCO*, 45 (6), p. 265-277. Available from: http://www.ebscohost.com [Accessed: 16 June 2015].

Williams, P. (2007). Medication errors. *Jr Coll Physicians Edinb*, 37 (4), pp. 343 – 346.

Wilson, R., et al., (1999). An Analysis of the causes of adverse events from the quality in Australian health care study. *Med J Aust, 170* (9), pp. 411 – 415.

World Health Organization. (2010). *Nursing and Midwifery Services*, Geneva, Switzerland: World Health Organization.

In: Investigating Patient Safety
Editor: Gloria Hale
ISBN: 978-1-53617-344-4
© 2020 Nova Science Publishers, Inc.

Chapter 5

AIR EMBOLISM AND HYPOTHERMIA ASSOCIATED WITH INTRAVENOUS FLUID THERAPY: RISK MANAGEMENT CONSIDERATIONS

Nickolas A. MacDougall[1], BS
and Mark E. Comunale[2], MD
[1]The Department of Anesthesiology, Arrowhead Regional Medical Center, Colton, California, US
[2]Loma Linda University, School of Medicine (M.E.C. and N.M.) and The Patient Safety Program, Arrowhead Regional Medical Center, Colton, California, US

ABSTRACT

Objective: Venous air embolism and hypothermia are serious and potential consequences of intravenous fluid therapy. Many patient populations may have increased risk of morbidly and mortality associated with these events. The risk management and financial impact of hospital acquired air embolism and hypothermia justifies active programs aimed at prevention. Devices used to mediate the risk of hypothermia may be sources of air embolism, making the presence of safety devices preventing infusion of air necessary.

Data Sources: The Medline publication library was used for initial literature identification.

Study Selection: A Medline publication search was conducted using keywords; air embolism, hypothermia, infusion device, inline, microbubble, transfusion cost, perioperative, prehospital, medicolegal cost.

Data Extraction and Synthesis: Publications with primary content focus of venous air embolism and hypothermia was selected for reviewed.

Conclusion: Inline fluid warming devices must employ the safest technology to ensure patients are not exposed to additional risks during active warming of infused fluids.

INTRODUCTION

Intravenous fluid (IVF) therapy is indicated in a wide variety of settings and pathologies for the purposes of volume resuscitation, maintenance, replacement and redistribution [1]. Fluid delivery rates may be categorized as high-flow (active, rapid, pressurized delivery) or low-flow (passive, slow, gravity driven delivery). In patients requiring rapid volume replacement, high-flow delivery systems are preferred, but have special risks associated with normal use. The majority of hospital and prehospital IVF therapy is delivered via low-flow delivery. Indications for prehospital IVF therapy are no different from hospital indications, but earlier access and IVF administration are associated with better patient outcomes [2, 3]. Prehospital IVF administration has recently been shown to significantly decrease in-hospital mortality in trauma patients [2]. Others have shown decreased risk of hospital mortality with prehospital IVF resuscitation in patients with severe sepsis [3]. Considering the widespread application of and number of patients receiving IVF, understanding IVF administration risks and mitigation strategies is essential for practitioners.

IVF infusion carries two significant and preventable negative outcomes: infusion-associated venous air embolism and hypothermia. Venous air embolism events are associated with both peripheral and central venous infusions, have high potential for iatrogenic morbidity and mortality [4, 5], and are preventable [6, 7]. Hypothermia contributes to negative surgical outcomes, decreased patient satisfaction, is not uncommon in the hospital and emergency medical services setting, and may be induced or worsened by infusion of cold fluids (<36°C) [8-11]. Successful prophylactic treatment with warmed IVF has been shown successful for maintaining normothermia in hypothermia susceptible patients [12, 13]. Effectively preventing both of these infusion-associated sequelae has traditionally been difficult as they are mutually exclusive in source and consequence to patients.

METHODS

Literature review using Medline database was conducted with combinations of search terms; air embolism, hypothermia, infusion device, inline, microbubble, transfusion cost, perioperative, prehospital, medicolegal cost. Identified publications were assessed for applicability to venous air embolism or hypothermia, then included or excluded. No Institutional Review Board approval was applied for or required, as there were no human subjects involved.

AIR EMBOLI AND MICROBUBBLES

Air embolism has been a Joint Commission reportable sentinel event since 1995 [4]. The incidence of symptomatic air embolism has been reported to occur at a rate of 2% [14]. Recommendations for prevention have been developed based on reviews of venous air embolism (VAE) events and their associated causes [4-6, 15, 16]. Yet, reports of sometimes deadly and preventable VAE persist [17-19].

VAE associated with central venous catheters (CVC) are the most commonly described cause of air embolism, are traditionally associated with catheter insertion or removal [4-6], and have reported mortality ranging from 23% to 50% [14-16]. However, an alarming proportion of CVC air embolism events occur at times other than catheter insertion and removal. The Pennsylvania Patient Safety Authority's review of CVC associated VAE events noted that up to 17% of such events occurred at times associated with fluid infusion [5]. In a separate review of CVC associated VAE, Heckmann et al. found 54% of events were caused by line disconnection during fluid infusion [15].

Instances of infusion related VAE are not limited to CVC, but have also been reported with less invasive infusion methods. Although less prevalent in the literature, multiple reports demonstrating VAE events during gravity drip peripheral IV infusions exist [20-25]. In most instances, the source of air was line disconnection, improperly primed tubing or air entrainment during changing of collapsible fluid bags. In addition to human error, there is evidence that standard gravity IV infusion results in formation of gas bubbles in the infusion line, which travel to the patient. When studying incidence of venous gas bubbles, Groell et al. found 4.3% of patients with peripheral IVs had detectable air emboli in the pulmonary trunk, right atrium or right ventricle [7]. Non-laminar flow, related to flow rate, length and diameter of tubing has been shown to create gas bubbles in infusion lines [4, 26, 27]. Infusion of warmed IVF to normothermic temperatures causes outgassing and formation of bubbles in infusion lines which may be infused into patients [14, 28, 29].

Microbubbles are small gas bubbles that typically enter venous circulation via infusion from an extracorporeal line [4, 27, 30]. While there is no consensus for defining microbubble size because of the dynamic cycle of microbubble aggregation into larger potentially harmful gas emboli then degradation back into microbubbles [4, 27, 30], they are generally defined as gas bubbles ranging from 3µm to 500µm [31-35].

Intravascular microbubble aggregation into larger gas bubbles capable of occluding flow represents the most acute pathology concern. However, secondary mechanisms of microbubble-induced tissue damage include: direct capillary endothelial damage causing increased vascular permeability and interstitial fluid accumulation [27, 36, 37], potentiation of neutrophil mediated inflammatory response via microvascular contact [27, 38], complement activation in response to gas/blood interface, [27, 39, 40, 41], and clotting system activation by sequestering platelets through aggregation and increased production of thrombin [42-45].

Several factors affect the degree of morbidly and mortality of VAE events. These are patient size/age, volume of air infused, location of vascular injection, location of air embolus seating, and speed of injection [4-6, 15, 16, 24, 27, 30]. Patients with anatomical variations allowing communication between venous and arterial circulation are most at risk. Paradoxical air embolism (PAE) is a well described phenomenon characterized by venous gas emboli causing proximal ischemic lesions to tissues supplied by arterial flow [46-50]. In most cases, patients were found to have right-to-left cardiac shunt through a patent foramen ovale (PFO), allowing gas emboli to bypass lung filtration. The prevalence of individuals with PFOs is between 10% and 40%, with 25% being the most commonly cited value [5, 51-53]. This mechanism of PAE is particularly concerning in neonates and pediatric patients because of their higher prevalence of PFOs and greater potential for harm with smaller air volumes [27]. A secondary PAE source is via non-cardiac right-to-left shunts such as intrapulmonary arteriovenous shunts (IPAVS) [54]. When evaluating healthy adults at rest, Laurie et al. detected IPAVS in 100% of their participants at variable Fi_{O2} [55]. PAEs have the potential to affect any organ with variable harm; as evident through reports of air emboli localizing in the coronary vasculature causing variable sequelae [56, 57] and well described cerebral ischemic events resulting from PAEs [15, 58-61]. There may also be a mechanism for so-called retrograde cerebral VAE, possibly resulting from jugular valve insufficiency, that does not require any right-to-left shunting and may cause significant adverse neurological outcomes [61-66]. Providers, risk managers, and hospitals should consider interventions to reduce patient exposure to VAEs, especially considering the multiple mechanisms for these events to cause negative adverse patient outcomes.

VAE FISCAL AND RISK MANAGEMENT CONSIDERATIONS

In 2008, the total cost of reported and preventable air embolism events was $8,299,000 with each event costing an average of $26,100 (n=318) [67]. This figure measures only the cost of care and treatment for the air embolism injury. Reported rates of VAEs caused by medical errors range from 78% to >90% [68, 69]. A review of closed claims for VAEs associated with central access devices identified median payments of $517,000, ranging from $304,000 to $1,076,000, with 75% of events resulting in death [70]. Additionally, 75% of these events occurred during CVC use (likely infusion), not insertion or removal. Another review of closed claims for VAE associated with peripheral intravenous catheters identified median payouts of $325,000, ranging from $25,800 to $4,120,000, with 50% of paid claims being associated with death [71]. Most of these VAE events resulted from air in autologous blood product infusion bags.

HYPOTHERMIA IN VARIOUS SETTINGS

Hypothermia, typically defined as a core body temperature less than 36°C, is not uncommon in the healthcare setting and carries established increases in negative outcomes. Physiologic consequences of hypothermia are increased infection rates [72, 73], coagulopathy [74], increased shivering causing increased O_2 consumption [75], hemodynamic instability and increased risk of mortality [10]. Inadvertent surgical hypothermia is known to increase risk of morbid cardiac events by 55% [10]. Perioperative hypothermia significantly increases PACU recovery time [76, 77], post-operative hospital stay, and wound healing time [78]. Prehospital hypothermia may be an independent risk factor for death and is associated with increased transfusion occurrence [79, 80].

Hypothermia may result from various sources depending on the particular patient environment. Perioperative hypothermia is typically attributed to anesthetic-induced thermal regulation dysfunction, surface exposure, and cold irrigation and infusion fluids [12, 81]. In the prehospital setting, up to two thirds of trauma patients may arrive hypothermic to emergency departments (ED) [82]. However, this may be a significant underrepresentation of hypothermia prevalence in trauma patients. Upon query of 3190 consecutive patients recently admitted to our institution's ED with traumatic injury, 79% demonstrated admission temperatures below 37°C [83]. This may result from shock, environmental exposure, and/or infusion of fluids [82, 84]. In a recent prospective study, ambient temperature correlated with administrated IVF temperatures causing the authors to suggest EDs discontinue and replace non-warmed IVF initiated by EMS [85]. Others have reported that prehospital administration of 250mL of IVF at room temperature (23.5°C) results in average ED arrival temperatures of 35.5°C [84]. Despite the frequency of hypothermia and it's consequences, strategies for mitigating hypothermia's effects may be easy to implement.

Regardless of setting, infusion of "cold" fluids (~23°C) can initiate and worsen hypothermia [11]. Conversely, warmed fluids may be used to halt, reverse and prophylactically treat hypothermia in hospital and prehospital setting [11-13, 84, 86]. Although reversal of hypothermia with administration of infused fluids alone is difficult and may require large volumes [87], successful reversal has been demonstrated [11]. Thus, focusing on prevention and maintenance of normothermia seems prudent. The administration of 600mL to 700mL of warm fluid (41°C) has been shown to significantly reduce the occurrence of perioperative hypothermia in preoperatively normothermic patients [13]. Yokoyama et al. found during Cesarean delivery infusion of 700mL IVF at 41°C maintained patient normothermia, significantly increased baby APGAR score, and umbilical arterial pH [86]. Prehospital infusion of warmed fluids (averaging 32.5°C) also has been shown to maintain normothermia [84].

An additional rational for administration of warmed fluids is increasing patient comfort and possibly satisfaction of care. Evaluation of patient comfort in various settings has demonstrated patient preference and increased comfort with administration of warmed IVF [8, 9, 84]. Independent of the environment, administration of warmed fluids should always be considered preferential to decrease risk of hypothermia, optimize outcomes and increase patient comfort.

HYPOTHERMIA FISCAL IMPACT

There is little primary data on the total direct costs of hypothermia in healthcare, however estimations for treatment of known sequelae have been described [88-92]. Independent of setting, even mild hypothermia (1°C) can significantly increase transfusion risk [80, 93, 94]. In patients presenting to the ED with temperatures <36°C, Klauke et al. found significantly increased risk for transfusion and an increase of 1.3units of PRBCs transfused, for patients requiring transfusion [79]. In 2011, United States PRBC acquisition costs averaged $225.42 per unit [89]. This value does not describe total costs of activities and overhead associated with transfusion, which have been calculated to cost some U.S. hospitals between $726.05 and $1183.32 per PRBC unit [90]. Perioperative hypothermia has been associated with increases in hospital length of stay by 2.6 to 9.3 days depending on type of procedure performed [78, 91]. According to 2014 data from the U.S. Healthcare Cost and Utilization Project, the cost of non-ICU surgical hospitalization was $3780 per day [92]. The corresponding cost of non-ICU medical hospitalization was $1854 per day [92]. Hypothermia is a pervasive problem in the prehospital and hospital setting, leads to increases in transfusion risk and requirement, increased mortality, increases in costs via length of stay, and in most instances, is preventable.

VAE, Hypothermia and Healthcare Quality

Considering the additional costs and potential penalties associated with air embolism and hypothermia, clinicians and institutions charged with the care of susceptible populations have a vested interest in prevention. VAE and hypothermia risk management recommendations promote education to increase awareness of risk factors [4, 5] and use of devices that include alarming and interventional safety features [95]. Institutional initiatives aimed at preventing care-acquired hypothermia and iatrogenic air embolism may satisfy several Medicare Quality Programs dictating reimbursements. Some of these directly related programs may include the Hospital-Acquired Condition Reduction Program (HAC), Value Based Purchasing Program (VBP), 30-day Readmission Reduction Program (RRP), and Serious Reportable Events (SRE). HAC, VBP, and RRP programs each carry reimbursement-based penalties for performance ranging from 1% to 3% of all hospital Medicare claims. In the case of SREs, injuries from VAEs result in zero reimbursement for SRE-related services.

Warming Infusion Devices: Effectiveness, Cost and Safety

On demand IVF warming, from ambient to body temperature during infusion requires one of several infusion warming devices, each with distinguishing risks, costs and efficacy. When implementing a normothermia program, there are several issues users and hospitals should consider. Infusion devices must be intrinsically safe by not increasing collateral risks of infusion such as VAE, must employ safe warming technology, and must protect the patient from other iatrogenic risks. Whether these devices be intended for the prehospital or hospital setting, they must effectively warm and deliver normothermic fluids to the patient under variable conditions. Finally, the device must be cost effective, reliable and sufficiently robust to be deployed anywhere within a care system.

Devices that attenuate the risk of VAE, including VAE caused by "outgassing" during warming [14, 28, 29], should be considered preferentially to more hazardous devices lacking air elimination or detection functions. Devices utilizing a 'water bath' to warm infusion fluids have leaked causing flow of recirculating fluid into the infusion path [96, 97]. In the case of one such device, the recirculating fluid which has the potential to be infused into the patient is either 0.3% Hydrogen Peroxide in distilled water, distilled water, or 35% Isopropyl Alcohol in distilled water [98]. In addition to the risks of infusing any one of these harmful preparations of recirculating fluid, proper upkeep of these recirculating fluids requires service personnel to perform maintenance as frequently as every 30 days [98]. In our opinion, the risk of harm from this device failure and cost of maintenance prohibit consideration of these devices for use.

The ability to effectively deliver appropriately warmed fluids to the patient is an important distinction from simply warming fluids. A great deal of heat is lost during flow of warmed fluids from a warming device to the vascular access site, causing hypothermic fluid infusion into the patient [99-101]. Close-to-patient warming is an effective strategy for combating effects of heat loss through IV tubing [100]. In addition to delivery of crystalloid fluids, IVF warming devices are used to warm and infuse otherwise cold (4°C storage temperature) blood products, making appropriate thermal regulation of fluids a concern for consideration. During transfusion, normothermic delivery of RBCs facilitates normal oxygen delivery via stability of the oxyhemoglobin disassociation curve. RBC hemolytic sensitivity to temperatures within one degree of normothermia [102] and decreases in RBC enzymatic activity at slightly hyperthermic temperatures suggests the importance of precise temperature regulation during heating [103]. Thus, devices that employ mechanisms to ensure delivery of properly warmed fluids to the patient should be preferred.

Table 1. Features vs Inline Fluid Warmers by Manufacturer

		Smith's Medical Hotline® HL-50	3M Ranger™	BD Enflow®	Belmont Buddy™ 2	Clinical Effect
Heating Technology		Indirect Recirculating Solution	Direct Dry Heating	Direct Dry Heating	Direct Dry Heating	Direct Dry Heating Eliminates Risk of Infused Recirculating Fluids [96-98]
		Jacketed Fluid Path	Warms Relatively Distant from Patient	Close to Patient Heating	Close to Patient Heating	Cooling of Infused Fluids Occurs During Flow from Device to Patient; Warming as Close to the Patient as Possible Reduces Fluid Cooling [99-101]
		Up to 4min to Set Point of Recirculating Fluid	~2min to Set Point	~1min to Set Point	<1min to Set Point	Quicker Fluid Warming Time Reduces Time to Normothermic Fluid Administration
		Recirculating Fluid Set Point (41°C ± 0.1°C)	Adjustable Infused Fluid Set Point (33°C-41°C)	Adjustable Infused Fluid Set Point (38°C-42°C ± 2°C)	Infused Fluid Set Point (38°C ± 2°C)	Reduction in Temperature variation around normothermia provides adequate warming and reduced risk of RBC thermal injury [102, 103]
Air Removal Safety Features		Optional Air Venting	Optional Air Venting	None	Standard, Integral, and Automatic Air Removal	Heated Fluids "Outgassing" Harmful Pockets of Air. Air Removal Provides a Necessary Level of Safety.
Design Considerations		Non-transportable, Relatively Heavy Weight (11lbs.), Requires Monthly Maintenance	Non-transportable, Light Weight (7.4lbs.), Low Maintenance	Transportable, Compact, Light Weight (4.5lbs.), Low Maintenance	Transportable, Compact, Light Weight (6.5lbs.), Low Maintenance	Applicability to various Care Settings, Mobility, and Ease of Maintenance Provides Effective Use, Safety and Reliability

Finally, a desirable feature of fluid warming devices is related to the ability to function reliably anywhere care is rendered. Valuable features include the ability to function with or without AC power in both the prehospital setting and during transportation of patients within a hospital, and the physical size of the device and resulting impact of its presence in the work environment. In this instance, devices that are not bulky or cumbersome may be integrated more seamlessly into daily care delivery. Table 1 represents some of these features in commonly used fluid warmers in the hospital and prehospital setting.

DISCUSSION

Three circumstances dictate the necessity for an active program focused on mitigating risk of VAE. First, the prevalence of PFOs, the likelihood that many patients may have the potential to form IPAVS, the possibility for retrograde venous embolism and the high potential for severe adverse patient outcomes when air embolism events occur. Second, the widespread use of IV therapy in the hospital and prehospital setting. Third, Medicare Quality Programs, which dictate Medicare reimbursements, provide a financial incentive for hospitals to reduce instances of VAE in their patients. An important detail to emphasize is that injuries secondary to VAE, a Serious Reportable Event, which receive no reimbursement for care related to these events.

When evaluating case reports of infusion related VAE, a common theme becomes clear: there was no use or mention of air detecting/alarming infusion safety devices being used [17-25]. Recommen-dations for use of such devices has been advocated in the literature repeatedly, however widespread dissemination of air detecting/alarming infusion devices is not observed in the hospital or prehospital setting [4, 5, 24, 95, 104]. Since many infusion related VAEs occur via line disconnection or improperly primed lines, distally placed air detection/elimination devices are currently recommended [95]. Devices capable of warming IVF to normothermic ranges are a viable option for limiting complications of both environmental and infusion related hypothermia.

CONCLUSION

Inline warming devices and air detection devices typically take up the same IV tubing real estate and can be difficult to set up and safely manage together. Integrated inline IV warming devices and air elimination devices achieve both desired functions in a small, safe, and easily manageable unit. In conclusion, managing air embolism and hypothermia risks associated with intravenous infusion therapy can be achieved in part by selection of infusion equipment designed to properly warm fluid and blood products and to detect/eliminate air within the system. Products that perform such functions and can be deployed as close to the patient as possible should be considered as part of any infusion therapy risk mitigation program.

REFERENCES

[1] National Clinical Guideline Centre (UK). *Intravenous Fluid Therapy in Adults in Hospital.* (2013). Available from: https://www.nice.org.uk/guidance/CG174?UNLID=965849685201711974425.

[2] Hampton DA, Fabricant LJ, Differding J, et al. Prehospital intravenous fluid is associated with increased survival in trauma patients. *J Trauma Acute Care Surg.* 2013; 75(1):S9–S15.

[3] Seymour CW, Cooke CR, Heckbert SR, et al. Prehospital intravenous access and fluid resuscitation in severe sepsis: an observational cohort study. *Crit Care.* 2014; 18:533.

[4] Cook LS. Infusion-related air embolism. *J Infus Nurs.* 2013 Jan-Feb; 36(1):26-36. doi: 10.1097/NAN.0b013e318279a804.

[5] Feil M. Reducing Risk of Air Embolism Associated with Central Venous Access Devices. *Pennsylvania Patient Safety Advisory*. 2012; 9. 58-64.
[6] Kusminsky RE. Complications of Central Venous Catheterization. *J Am Coll Surg*. 2007 Apr; 204(4):681-96.
[7] Groell R, Schaffler GJ, Rienmueller R. The Peripheral Intravenous Cannula: A Cause of Venous Air Embolism. *Am J Med Sci*. 1997 Nov; 314(5):300-2.
[8] Self WH, White SJ, McNaughton CD, et al. Warming intravenous fluids for improved patient comfort in the emergency department: a pilot crossover randomized controlled trial. *West J Emerg Med*. 2013 Sep; 14(5):542-6.
[9] Youn AM, Hsu TM. Heated carrier fluids in decreasing propofol injection pain: a randomized, controlled trial. *Korean J Anesthesiol*. 2017 Feb; 70(1):33-38.
[10] Frank SM, Fleisher LA, Breslow MJ, et al. Perioperative maintenance of normothermia reduces the incidence of morbid cardiac events. A randomized clinical trial. *JAMA*. 1997 Apr 9; 277(14):1127-34.
[11] Barthel ER, Pierce JR. Steady-state and time-dependent thermodynamic modeling of the effect of intravenous infusion of warm and cold fluids. *J Trauma Acute Care Surg*. 2012 Jun; 72(6):1590-600.
[12] Campbell G, Alderson P, Smith AF, et al. Warming of intravenous and irrigation fluids for preventing inadvertent perioperative hypothermia. *Cochrane Database Syst Rev*. 2015 Apr 13; (4):CD009891.
[13] Kim G, Kim MH, Lee SM, et al. Effect of pre-warmed intravenous fluids on perioperative hypothermia and shivering after ambulatory surgery under monitored anesthesia care. *J Anesth*. 2014 Dec; 28(6):880-5.
[14] Erkin Y, Taşdöğen A, Gönüllü E. Is there risk of emboli during infusion with line type blood-liquid warmers? *Braz J Anesthesiol*. 2013 Sep-Oct; 63(5):389-92.

[15] Heckmann JG, Lang CJ, Kindler K, et al. Neurologic manifestations of cerebral air embolism as a complication of central venous catheterization. *Crit Care Med.* 2000 May; 28(5):1621-5.

[16] Kashuk JL, Penn I. Air embolism after central venous catheterization. *Surg Gynecol Obstet.* 1984 Sep; 159(3):249-52.

[17] Suwanpratheep, A., & Siriussawakul, A. Inadvertent Venous Air Embolism from Pressure Infuser Bag Confirmed by Transesophageal Echocardiography. *J Anesth Clin Res.* 2011; 02(10).

[18] Toung TJ, Rossberg MI, Hutchins GM. Volume of air in a lethal venous air embolism. *Anesthesiology.* 2001 Feb;94(2):360-1.

[19] Adhikary GS, Massey SR. Massive air embolism: a case report. *J Clin Anesth.* 1998 Feb; 10(1):70-2.

[20] Agarwal SS, Kumar L, Chavali KH, et al. Fatal venous air embolism following intravenous infusion. *J Forensic Sci.* 2009 May; 54(3):682-4.

[21] Sowell MW, Lovelady CL, Brogdon BG, et al. Infant death due to air embolism from peripheral venous infusion. *J Forensic Sci.* 2007 Jan; 52(1):183-8.

[22] Wald M, Kirchner L, Lawrenz K, et al. Fatal air embolism in an extremely low birth weight infant: can it be caused by intravenous injections during resuscitation? *Intensive Care Med.* 2003 Apr; 29(4):630-3.

[23] Bakan M, Topuz U, Esen A, et al. Inadvertent venous air embolism during cesarean section: Collapsible intravenous fluid bags without self-sealing outlet have risks. *Case report. Braz J Anesthesiol.* 2013 Jul-Aug; 63(4):362-5.

[24] Laskey AL, Dyer C, Tobias JD. Venous air embolism during home infusion therapy. *Pediatrics.* 2002 Jan; 109(1):E15.

[25] Levy I, Mosseri R, Garty B. Peripheral intravenous infusion--another cause of air embolism. *Acta Paediatr.* 1996 Mar; 85(3):385-6.

[26] Hartmannsgruber MW, Gravenstein N. Very limited air elimination capability of the level 1 fluid warmer. *J Clin Anesth.* 1997 May; 9(3):233-5.

[27] Barak M, Katz Y. Microbubbles: pathophysiology and clinical implications. *Chest.* 2005 Oct; 128(4):2918-32.

[28] Varga C, Luria I, Gravenstein N. Intravenous Air: The Partially Invisible Phenomenon. *Anesth Analg.* 2016 Nov; 123(5):1149-1155.

[29] Woon S, Talke P. Amount of air infused to patient increases as fluid flow rates decrease when using the Hotline HL-90 fluid warmer. *J Clin Monit Comput.* 1999 May; 15(3-4):149-52.

[30] Barak M, Nakhoul F, Katz Y. Pathophysiology and clinical implications of microbubbles during hemodialysis. *Semin Dial.* 2008 May-Jun; 21(3):232-8.

[31] Newland RF, Baker RA, Mazzone AL, et al. Should Air Bubble Detectors Be Used to Quantify Microbubble Activity during Cardiopulmonary Bypass? *J Extra Corpor Technol.* 2015 Sep; 47(3):174-9.

[32] Keshavarzi G, Simmons A, Yeoh G, et al. Effectiveness of microbubble removal in an airtrap with a free surface interface. *J Biomech.* 2015 May 1; 48(7):1237-40.

[33] Sobolewski P, Kandel J, Klinger AL, et al. Air bubble contact with endothelial cells in vitro induces calcium influx and IP3-dependent release of calcium stores. *Am J Physiol Cell Physiol.* 2011 Sep; 301(3):C679-86.

[34] Suzuki A, Eckmann DM. Embolism bubble adhesion force in excised perfused microvessels. *Anesthesiology.* 2003 Aug; 99(2):400-8.

[35] Abu-Omar Y, Balacumaraswami L, Pigott DW, et al. Solid and gaseous cerebral microembolization during off-pump, on-pump, and open cardiac surgery procedures. *J Thorac Cardiovasc Surg.* 2004 Jun; 127(6):1759-65.

[36] Albertine KH, Wiener-Kronish JP, Koike K, et al. Quantification of damage by air emboli to lung microvessels in anesthetized sheep. *J Appl Physiol Respir Environ Exerc Physiol.* 1984 Nov; 57(5):1360-8.

[37] Ohkuda K, Nakahara K, Binder A, et al. Venous air emboli in sheep: reversible increase in lung microvascular permeability. *J Appl Physiol Respir Environ Exerc Physiol.* 1981 Oct; 51(4):887-94.

[38] Ohkuda K, Nakahara K, Weidner WJ, et al. Lung fluid exchange after uneven pulmonary artery obstruction in sheep. *Circ Res. 1978* Aug; 43(2):152-61.

[39] Ward CA, Koheil A, McCullough D, et al. Activation of complement at plasma-air or serum-air interface of rabbits. *J Appl Physiol (1985).* 1986 May; 60(5):1651-8.

[40] Jacob HS. Complement-mediated leucoembolization: a mechanism of tissue damage during extracorporeal perfusions, myocardial infarction and in shock--a review. *Q J Med.* 1983 Summer; 52 (207):289-96.

[41] Nossum V, Hjelde A, Bergh K, et al. Anti-C5a monoclonal antibodies and pulmonary polymorphonuclear leukocyte infiltration--endothelial dysfunction by venous gas embolism. *Eur J Appl Physiol.* 2003 May;89(3-4):243-8.

[42] Malik AB, Johnson A, Tahamont MV. Mechanisms of lung vascular injury after intravascular coagulation. *Ann N Y Acad Sci.* 1982; 384:213-34.

[43] Eckmann DM, Diamond SL. Surfactants attenuate gas embolism-induced thrombin production. *Anesthesiology.* 2004 Jan; 100(1):77-84.

[44] Thorsen T, Dalen H, Bjerkvig R, et al. Transmission and scanning electron microscopy of N2 microbubble-activated human platelets in vitro. *Undersea Biomed Res.* 1987 Jan; 14(1):45-58.

[45] Warren BA, Philp RB, Inwood MJ. The ultrastructural morphology of air embolism: platelet adhesion to the interface and endothelialdamage. *Br J Exp Pathol.* 1973 Apr; 54(2):163-72.

[46] Gronert GA, Messick JM Jr, Cucchiara RF, et al. Paradoxical air embolism from a patent foramen ovale. *Anesthesiology.* 1979 Jun; 50(6):548-9.

[47] Michel L, Poskanzer DC, McKusick KA, et al. Fatal paradoxical air embolism to the brain: complication of central venous catheterization. *JPEN J Parenter Enteral Nutr.* 1982 Jan-Feb; 6(1):68-70.

[48] Jacobsen WK, Briggs BA, Mason LJ. Paradoxical air embolism associated with a central total parenteral nutrition catheter. *Crit Care Med.* 1983 May; 11(5):388-9.

[49] Eichhorn V, Bender A, Reuter DA. Paradoxical air embolism from a central venous catheter. *Br J Anaesth.* 2009 May;102(5):717-8.

[50] Han SS, Kim SS, Hong HP, et al. Massive paradoxical air embolism in brain occurring after central venous catheterization: a casereport. *J Korean Med Sci.* 2010 Oct; 25(10):1536-8.

[51] American Heart Association. *Patent Formen Ovale (PFO).* 2017. Accessed February 2017. Available at http://www.heart.org/HEARTORG/Conditions/More/CardiovascularConditionsofChildhood/Patent-Foramen-Ovale-PFO_UCM_469590_Article.jsp#.WdLs96OZN1M.

[52] Fisher DC, Fisher EA, Budd JH, et al. The incidence of patent foramen ovale in 1,000 consecutive patients. A contrast transesophagealechocardiography study. *Chest.* 1995 Jun; 107(6):1504-9.

[53] Lynch JJ, Schuchard GH, Gross CM, et al. Prevalence of right-to-left atrial shunting in a healthy population: detection by Valsalva maneuvercontrast echocardiography. *Am J Cardiol.* 1984 May 15; 53(10):1478-80.

[54] Siegenthaler N, Giraud R, Courvoisier DS, et al. Effects of acute hemorrhage on intrapulmonary shunt in a pig model of acute respiratory distress-like syndrome. *BMC Pulm Med.* 2016 Apr 26; 16(1):59.

[55] Laurie SS, Yang X, Elliott JE, et al. Hypoxia-induced intrapul-monary arteriovenous shunting at rest in healthy humans. *J Appl Physiol (1985).* 2010 Oct; 109(4):1072-9.

[56] Lee HY, Yoo SM. A case of paradoxical air embolism in the coronary artery through a patent foramen ovaledemonstrated by coronary CT angiography. *Clin Imaging.* 2013 Jan-Feb;37(1):167-9.

[57] Kazimirko DN, Beam WB, Saleh K, et al. Beware of positive pressure: coronary artery air embolism following percutaneous lung biopsy. *Radiol Case Rep.* 2016 Sep 17; 11(4):344-347.

[58] Bartolini L, Burger K. Pearls & oy-sters: cerebral venous air embolism after central catheter removal: too much air can kill. *Neurology.* 2015 Mar 31; 84(13):e94-6.

[59] Brockmeyer J, Johnson EK. Cerebral air embolism following removal of central venous catheter. *Mil Med.* 2011 Feb;176(2):i.

[60] Opeskin K, Burke MP, Lynch M. Cerebral air embolism due to disconnection of a central venous catheter. *J Clin Neurosci.* 1998 Oct;5(4):469-71.

[61] Schlimp CJ, Loimer T, Rieger M, et al. Pathophysiological mechanism and immediate treatment of retrograde cerebral venous air embolism. *Intensive Care Med.* 2006 Jun; 32(6):945.

[62] Fracasso T, Karger B, Schmidt PF, et al. Retrograde venous cerebral air embolism from disconnected central venous catheter: an experimental model. *J Forensic Sci.* 2011 Jan; 56 Suppl 1:S101-4.

[63] Schlimp CJ, Loimer T, Rieger M, et al. The potential of venous air embolism ascending retrograde to the brain. *J Forensic Sci.* 2005 Jul; 50(4):906-9.

[64] Brouns R, De Surgeloose D, Neetens I, et al. Fatal venous cerebral air embolism secondary to a disconnected central venous catheter. *Cerebrovasc Dis.* 2006; 21(3):212-4.

[65] Schlimp CJ, Lederer W. Factors facilitating retrograde cerebral venous air embolism. *J Child Neurol.* 2008 Aug;23(8):973;

[66] Nedelmann M, Pittermann P, Gast KK, et al. Involvement of jugular valve insufficiency in cerebral venous air embolism. *J Neuroimaging.* 2007 Jul; 17(3):258-60.

[67] Van Den Bos J, Rustagi K, Gray T, et al. The $17.1 billion problem: the annual cost of measurable medical errors. *Health Aff (Millwood).* 2011 Apr; 30(4):596-603.

[68] Shreve J, Van Den Bos J, Gray T, et al. *The Economic Measurement of Medical Errors. Society of Actuaries.* 2010. Accessed March 2017. Available at https://www.soa.org/research-reports/2010/research-econ-measurement/

[69] Kandilov A, Dalton K, Coomer N. *Analysis report: estimating the incremental costs of hospital-acquired conditions (HACS).* (Prepared by RTI International under Contract No. 500-T00007.) Baltimore, MD: Centers for Medicare & Medicaid Services; 2011.

[70] Domino KB, Bowdle TA, Posner KL, et al. Injuries and liability related to central vascular catheters: a closed claims analysis. *Anesthesiology.* 2004 Jun; 100(6):1411-8.

[71] Bhananker SM, Liau DW, Kooner PK, et al. Liability related to peripheral venous and arterial catheterization: a closed claims analysis. *Anesth Analg.* 2009 Jul; 109(1):124-9.

[72] Haley RW, Culver DH, Morgan WM, et al. Identifying patients at high risk of surgical wound infection. A simple multivariate index of patientsusceptibility and wound contamination. *Am J Epidemiol.* 1985 Feb; 121(2):206-15.

[73] Culver DH, Horan TC, Gaynes RP, et al. Surgical wound infection rates by wound class, operative procedure, and patient risk index. National Nosocomial Infections Surveillance System. *Am J Med.* 1991 Sep 16; 91(3B):152S-157S.

[74] Lier H, Krep H, Schroeder S, et al. Preconditions of hemostasis in trauma: a review. The influence of acidosis, hypocalcemia, anemia, and hypothermia on functional hemostasis in trauma. *J Trauma.* 2008 Oct; 65(4):951-60.

[75] Frank SM, Fleisher LA, Olson KF, et al. Multivariate determinants of early postoperative oxygen consumption in elderly patients. Effects of shivering, body temperature, and gender. *Anesthesiology.* 1995 Aug; 83(2):241-9.

[76] Vaughan MS, Vaughan RW, Cork RC. Postoperative hypothermia in adults: relationship of age, anesthesia, and shivering to rewarming. *Anesth Analg.* 1981 Oct; 60(10):746-51.

[77] Lenhardt R, Marker E, Goll V, et al. Mild intraoperative hypothermia prolongs post-anesthetic recovery. *Anesthesiology.* 1997 Dec; 87(6):1318-23.

[78] Kurz A, Sessler DI, Lenhardt R. Perioperative normothermia to reduce the incidence of surgical-wound infection and shorten hospitalization. Study of Wound Infection and Temperature Group. *N Engl J Med.* 1996 May 9; 334(19):1209-15.

[79] Klauke N, Gräff I, Fleischer A, et al. Effects of prehospital hypothermia on transfusion requirements and outcomes: a

retrospectiveobservatory trial. *BMJ Open.* 2016 Mar 30; 6(3): e009913.

[80] Bukur M, Hadjibashi AA, Ley EJ, et al. Impact of prehospital hypothermia on transfusion requirements and outcomes. *J Trauma Acute Care Surg.* 2012 Nov; 73(5):1195-201.

[81] Comunale ME: Risk management considerations in surgical fluid management: the prevention of hypothermia and new advances in fluid warming technology. *Today's Ther Trends* 2000; 18: 87–95.

[82] Luna GK, Maier RV, Pavlin EG, et al. Incidence and effect of hypothermia in seriously injured patients. *J Trauma.* 1987 Sep; 27(9):1014-8.

[83] *ARMC Trauma Registry.* Query Dates 1/1/2016-12/31/2017. Accessed March 2017. Available from Trauma Services Department, Arrowhead Regional Medical Center, Colton, CA.

[84] Cassidy ES, Adkins CR, Rayl JH, et al. Evaluation of warmed intravenous fluids in the prehospital setting. *Air Med J.* 2001 Sep-Oct;20(5):25-6.

[85] Joslin J, Fisher A, Wojcik S, et al. A prospective evaluation of the contribution of ambient temperatures and transport times on infrared thermometry readings of intravenous fluids utilized in EMS patients. *Int J Emerg Med.* 2014 Dec 16;7(1):47.

[86] Yokoyama K, Suzuki M, Shimada Y, et al. Effect of administration of pre-warmed intravenous fluids on the frequency of hypothermiafollowing spinal anesthesia for Cesarean delivery. *J Clin Anesth.* 2009 Jun; 21(4):242-8.

[87] Gill BS, Cox CS Jr. Thermodynamic and logistic considerations for treatment of hypothermia. *Mil Med.* 2008 Aug; 173(8):743-8.

[88] Stubbs JR. Wrapping our arms around the cost of transfusion therapy. *Transfusion.* 2014 Feb; 54(2):259-62.

[89] Whitaker B. *The 2011 National Blood Collection and Utilization Survey Report.* (Survey Conducted by AABB Under Contract HHSP23320110008TC.) US Department of Health and Human Services. 2011 Available at https://www.aabb.org/research/hemovigilance/bloodsurvey/Documents/11-nbcus-report.pdf.

[90] Shander A, Hofmann A, Ozawa S, et al. Activity-based costs of blood transfusions in surgical patients at four hospitals. *Transfusion.* 2010 Apr; 50(4):753-65.

[91] Bush HL Jr, Hydo LJ, Fischer E, et al. Hypothermia during elective abdominal aortic aneurysm repair: the high price of avoidable morbidity. *J Vasc Surg.* 1995 Mar;21(3):392-400.

[92] HCUP Fast Stats. Healthcare Cost and Utilization Project (HCUP). *Agency for Healthcare Research and Quality,* Rockville, MD. 2016 Available at www.hcup-us.ahrq.gov/faststats/national/inpatient-trends.jsp?measure1=03&characteristic1=06&time1=10&measure2=04&characteristic2=06&time2=10&expansionInfoState=hide&dataTablesState=hide&definitionsState=hide&exportState.

[93] Sun Z, Honar H, Sessler DI, et al. Intraoperative core temperature patterns, transfusion requirement, and hospital duration in patients warmed with forced air. *Anesthesiology.* 2015 Feb; 122(2):276-85.

[94] Rajagopalan S, Mascha E, Na J, et al. The effects of mild perioperative hypothermia on blood loss and transfusion requirement. *Anesthesiology.* 2008 Jan; 108(1):71-7.

[95] The Joint Commission. Clinical Care Improvement Strategies: Preventing Air Embolism. *The Joint Commission Resources,* Chicago, IL; 2010 Accessed March 2017. Available at http://www.jcrinc.com/assets/1/14/ebpae10_sample_pages.pdf.

[96] Clarke PA, Thornton MJ. Failure of a water-bath design intravenous fluid warmer. *Can J Anaesth.* 2009 Nov; 56(11):876-7.

[97] Wilson S, Szerb J. Failure of an iv fluid warming device. *Can J Anaesth.* 2007 Apr; 54(4):324-5.

[98] OPERATOR'S MANUAL Level 1 HOTLINE®Blood and Fluid Warmer (HL-90). *Smith's Medical.* 2013. Accessed March 2017. Available at http://level1hotline.com/pdf/HL-90_4534005-GB%"20Rev-010_Print.pdf.

[99] Karlsen AM, Thomassen O, Vikenes BH, et al. Equipment to prevent, diagnose, and treat hypothermia: a survey of Norwegian pre-hospitalservices. *Scand J Trauma Resusc Emerg Med.* 2013 Aug 12;21:63.

[100] Faries G, Johnston C, Pruitt KM, et al. Temperature relationship to distance and flow rate of warmed i.v. fluids. *Ann Emerg Med.* 1991 Nov; 20(11):1198-200.

[101] Handrigan MT, Wright RO, Becker BM, et al. Factors and methodology in achieving ideal delivery temperatures for intravenous and lavage fluidin hypothermia. *Am J Emerg Med.* 1997 Jul; 15(4):350-3.

[102] Gershfeld NL, Murayama M. Thermal instability of red blood cell membrane bilayers: temperature dependence of hemolysis. *J Membr Biol.* 1988; 101(1):67-72.

[103] Marks RJ, Minty BD, White DC. Warming blood before transfusion. Does immersion warming change blood composition? *Anaesthesia.* 1985 Jun; 40(6):541-4.

[104] McCarthy CJ, Behravesh S, Naidu SG, et al. Air Embolism: Practical Tips for Prevention and Treatment. *J Clin Med.* 2016 Oct 31; 5(11). pii: E93.

INDEX

#

1st and 2nd generation human error models, 2, 9

A

access, 86, 122, 126, 130, 133
adults, 31, 125, 140
adverse effects, 45, 99, 110
adverse event, 3, 6, 7, 8, 27, 30, 60, 92, 93, 115, 119
advocacy, vii, x, 98, 99, 100, 101, 103, 104, 105, 113, 114, 115, 116, 117, 118
advocate, x, 98, 100, 103, 105, 113, 115
age, 44, 50, 104, 106, 125, 140
air embolism, xi, 121, 122, 123, 124, 125, 126, 129, 132, 133, 135, 137, 138, 139
allergy, 108, 109, 110, 111, 112, 118
antibiotic, 108, 109, 110, 111
arrest, 109, 111, 112
artery, 106, 107, 138
assessment, ix, 3, 22, 44, 60, 62, 72, 73, 80, 83, 84, 86, 87, 88, 89, 96, 111
attitudes, 4, 27, 42, 93, 99, 101, 102, 114

attribution, viii, 1, 4, 7, 10
audit, 17, 43, 70
auscultation, 45, 106, 109
autopsy, viii, 30, 32, 49, 60
awareness, 37, 41, 47, 51, 56, 129

B

bad apples theory, 2
bias, vii, ix, 30, 35, 37, 38, 40, 49, 52, 55, 56, 62, 63, 66
blood, 45, 106, 108, 109, 125, 126, 130, 133, 134, 142, 143
blood pressure, 45, 106, 109
brain, 14, 18, 137, 138, 139
burnout, 39, 46, 49, 58, 66, 67, 70

C

CAF, ix, 72, 73, 74, 75, 76, 77, 78, 79, 80, 83, 84, 85, 86, 87, 88, 89, 90, 96
cancer, 35, 41, 113
case study, 107, 110, 111, 112
catheter, 124, 137, 138, 139
causality, viii, 1, 7

challenges, 47, 100, 104
citizens, ix, 72, 73, 74, 75, 77, 81, 82
classification, 20, 34, 35
clinical diagnosis, 32, 48, 67, 68, 69
clinical examination, 36, 39, 40, 65, 106
closure, 37, 40, 44, 55, 56
cognitive biases, 46, 61, 63, 70
cognitive process, 10, 15, 19
common assessment framework, 72
communication, ix, 19, 30, 64, 88, 125
community, 25, 78, 99, 100
complement, 22, 125, 137
complexity, 7, 18, 43, 44
compliance, 102, 105, 107, 112, 117
cooperation, 19, 35, 88, 104
cost, xi, 30, 55, 122, 123, 126, 128, 130, 139, 141
critical thinking, 42, 47, 56, 61
criticism, viii, 1, 38
culture, x, 8, 30, 43, 50, 60, 76, 77, 84, 97, 101, 103, 106, 109, 114, 118
customers, ix, 72, 73, 77, 81, 82

D

data collection, 32, 36, 44, 51
data gathering, 36, 39, 49
depression, 39, 50, 59
detection, 130, 132, 133, 138
differential diagnosis, 35, 39, 44, 47
diseases, 35, 57, 70
distress, 66, 67, 138
diversity, 62, 84, 87

E

education, 12, 20, 39, 42, 48, 50, 68, 69, 96, 101, 102, 114, 129
emboli, 124, 125, 134, 136
embolism, xi, 121, 122, 123, 124, 125, 126, 129, 132, 133, 135, 137, 138, 139

emergency, 31, 32, 33, 34, 65, 108, 110, 123, 127, 134
employees, 7, 15, 20, 73, 78, 80, 81, 85, 88, 105
environment, 3, 13, 14, 15, 21, 34, 78, 127, 128
equipment, 3, 6, 13, 16, 133
ethics, v, vii, x, xi, 75, 84, 97, 98, 99, 100, 102, 105, 107, 112, 113, 114, 115, 117, 118
Europe, 73, 74, 80
European Union, 74, 75, 86, 87, 88
evidence, x, xi, 41, 42, 43, 45, 56, 66, 73, 83, 98, 99, 101, 107, 114, 124
execution, 5, 9, 14, 16
expertise, 37, 55, 68, 69

F

families, 103, 105, 110
financial, xi, 74, 82, 122, 132
fluid, vii, xi, 121, 122, 124, 125, 127, 130, 132, 133, 135, 136, 137, 141, 142
foramen, 125, 137, 138
foramen ovale, 125, 137, 138

G

Google, 44, 47, 53, 66, 67
Greece, 1, 26, 27, 28, 71, 91, 92, 93, 94
guidance, 73, 75, 133
guidelines, 43, 46, 102

H

health, viii, x, 22, 29, 30, 31, 34, 41, 43, 48, 58, 59, 60, 61, 66, 69, 70, 94, 97, 99, 100, 101, 103, 104, 105, 113, 114, 119
health care, viii, 22, 29, 30, 41, 69, 70, 99, 100, 113, 114, 119

Index

high reliability organizations theory, 2
history, 35, 36, 39, 40, 44, 45, 50, 53, 58, 65, 69, 108
human, vii, viii, ix, 1, 2, 3, 4, 5, 6, 7, 9, 10, 11, 12, 13, 14, 15, 16, 17, 18, 19, 20, 21, 22, 23, 24, 25, 60, 72, 77, 78, 81, 82, 101, 103, 112, 113, 123, 124, 137
human behavior, 9, 10, 14
human resources, ix, 72, 77, 78, 81, 82
hypothermia, vi, xi, 121, 122, 123, 126, 127, 128, 129, 133, 134, 140, 141, 142, 143

I

iatrogenic, viii, 29, 30, 31, 48, 53, 69, 123, 129
ideal(s), 22, 101, 103, 105, 113, 143
identification, xi, 3, 30, 31, 32, 84, 85, 107, 108, 111, 112, 115, 122
improvements, 31, 34, 75, 85
incidence, ix, 30, 31, 33, 61, 102, 123, 124, 134, 138, 140
individuals, 3, 11, 16, 17, 18, 19, 21, 22, 98, 103, 125
infusion device, xi, 122, 123, 129, 132
injuries, 31, 129, 132
injury/injuries, 31, 103, 126, 127, 129, 131, 132, 137
inline, vii, xi, 122, 123, 131, 133
interface, 35, 125, 136, 137
intervention, viii, 29, 104, 106, 107
intravenous, vi, xi, 109, 111, 121, 122, 126, 133, 134, 135, 136, 141, 142, 143
issues, 5, 39, 43, 80, 101, 102, 105, 107, 112, 129

L

laboratory tests, 44, 50, 53, 108
lead, x, 8, 10, 12, 14, 15, 35, 41, 72, 73, 77, 88, 106

leadership, ix, 72, 77, 85, 101
learning, ix, x, 3, 12, 39, 42, 44, 45, 49, 53, 58, 63, 72, 76, 78, 80, 85, 86, 98, 102, 116
lesions, 37, 106, 125

M

management, vii, xi, 3, 5, 19, 24, 25, 27, 42, 47, 64, 66, 76, 80, 86, 92, 96, 99, 101, 106, 118, 122, 129, 141
measurement, 57, 64, 84, 139
medical, x, 3, 5, 27, 30, 34, 36, 39, 42, 43, 45, 48, 50, 53, 59, 60, 61, 62, 63, 64, 65, 66, 67, 68, 69, 70, 92, 93, 96, 98, 101, 106, 107, 108, 109, 110, 112, 113, 116, 123, 126, 128, 139
medical error, x, 3, 5, 27, 30, 34, 59, 61, 62, 66, 67, 92, 93, 98, 110, 112, 113, 116, 126, 139
Medicare, 33, 61, 129, 132, 139
medicare reimbursement, 132
medication, viii, 27, 29, 93, 109, 110, 111, 112, 118
medicine, 24, 32, 34, 36, 41, 42, 45, 47, 49, 50, 60, 61, 62, 63, 64, 65, 66, 67, 68, 69, 101
medicolegal cost, xi, 122, 123
memory, 5, 14, 16, 17, 20, 46
methodology, 22, 24, 89, 143
microbubble, xi, 122, 123, 124, 125, 136, 137
models, 2, 5, 9, 10, 11, 12, 13, 14, 15, 18, 19, 20, 21, 25, 39, 41
morbidity, 113, 123, 142
mortality, viii, xi, 29, 36, 113, 122, 123, 124, 125, 126, 128

N

negative outcomes, 104, 123, 126

neglect, 37, 55, 59
Netherlands, 75, 76, 85
normal accident theories, 2
nurses, 100, 101, 103, 104, 110, 113, 114, 115, 117, 118, 119
nursing, 96, 99, 100, 101, 102, 104, 105, 108, 109, 110, 111, 113, 114, 116, 117, 118

O

omission, 3, 4, 9, 14, 19, 35, 44, 53
operations, 11, 12, 25
oxygen, 45, 108, 130, 140

P

pain, 45, 106, 116, 134
parallel, 3, 17, 20
parents, 27, 93, 108, 109
pathology, 35, 56, 125
patient care, xi, 49, 66, 67, 98, 100, 102, 103, 104, 105, 107, 114
pattern recognition, 37, 38, 46, 55, 63
perioperative, xi, 122, 123, 126, 127, 128, 134, 140
physicians, 32, 33, 39, 40, 42, 43, 45, 46, 49, 61, 65, 66, 68, 70, 101
policy, 8, 35, 44, 70, 81, 89, 106, 107, 112, 114
population, 43, 113, 138
prehospital, xi, 122, 123, 126, 127, 128, 129, 132, 133, 140, 141
prevention, xi, 4, 9, 24, 30, 31, 42, 59, 94, 99, 103, 122, 123, 127, 129, 141
principles, vii, ix, 3, 7, 30, 43, 44, 48, 49, 50, 59, 72, 73, 76, 77, 78, 84, 86, 99, 100, 110
probability, 6, 8, 10, 11, 12, 13, 15, 18, 21, 36, 39, 44, 53, 54, 62
problem solving, 20, 41, 61, 64

problem-solving, 49, 51, 63, 69
professionals, x, 70, 97, 98, 100, 102, 104, 105, 107, 110, 111, 112, 113, 114
protection, 4, 103, 104

Q

quality, v, vii, x, xi, 1, 3, 5, 7, 13, 23, 24, 26, 27, 28, 39, 41, 60, 61, 72, 73, 74, 75, 76, 77, 79, 82, 83, 84, 86, 87, 88, 91, 92, 93, 94, 95, 96, 97, 98, 100, 101, 103, 104, 105, 106, 110, 112, 114, 115, 119, 129, 132, 142
quality in healthcare services, 72

R

RBC, 128, 130, 131
reasoning, ix, 30, 31, 35, 39, 41, 43, 45, 46, 48, 49, 50, 52, 55, 56, 61, 63, 66, 68, 69, 70
recognition, 38, 42, 52, 55, 78
recovery, 107, 126, 140
reliability, 2, 6, 11, 12, 13, 24, 25
requirement(s), 17, 24, 43, 74, 78, 110, 128, 140, 141, 142
researchers, 9, 47, 104
resources, ix, 4, 66, 72, 77, 78, 81, 82
respiratory rate, 45, 106, 109
response, 15, 17, 74, 103, 125
resuscitation, 117, 122, 133, 135
rights, 24, 100, 104, 110, 111, 113
risk(s), vii, x, xi, 3, 5, 21, 23, 24, 34, 43, 44, 53, 59, 97, 100, 103, 104, 107, 110, 113, 122, 125, 126, 128, 129, 130, 131, 132, 133, 134, 135, 140
risk factors, 44, 53, 59, 129
risk management, xi, 122, 129, 141

Index

S

safety, v, vii, viii, ix, x, xi, 3, 8, 10, 22, 23, 24, 25, 26, 27, 28, 29, 30, 31, 34, 40, 41, 42, 43, 47, 49, 59, 60, 61, 64, 71, 90, 91, 92, 93, 94, 95, 96, 97, 98, 99, 100, 101, 102, 103, 104, 105, 106, 107, 110, 111, 112, 113, 114, 116, 118, 121,122, 124, 129, 131, 132, 134
science, viii, xi, 2, 3, 7, 48, 66, 68, 98
security, 6, 8, 19
self-assessment, vii, ix, 72, 73, 74, 76, 79, 80, 83, 84, 85, 86, 88, 89
self-assessment of hospital, 72
sensitivity, 46, 109, 130
services, vii, x, 3, 8, 72, 73, 77, 82, 98, 123, 129
signs, 40, 45, 53, 54
social responsibility, ix, 72, 75, 78
society, ix, 72, 73, 74, 77, 82, 104
stakeholders, 75, 84, 85
state, 15, 19, 49, 55, 84, 89, 112, 134
stress, 39, 59, 70
structure, ix, 4, 8, 18, 72, 73, 78, 88
symptoms, 51, 53, 54

T

target, viii, 29, 43
techniques, ix, 3, 10, 11, 30, 33, 36, 38, 48, 73, 74
technology/technologies, vii, viii, xi, 15, 30, 37, 47, 69, 81, 113, 122, 129, 141
temperature, 45, 108, 126, 127, 129, 130, 140, 142, 143
testing, 33, 36, 42, 45, 56, 65, 66
textbooks, 46, 54, 56
theory-practice-gap, 98
therapy, xi, 108, 121, 122, 132, 133, 135, 141
time constraints, 34, 43, 46, 65
training, 23, 39, 44
transfusion, xi, 122, 123, 127, 128, 130, 140, 141, 142, 143
transfusion cost, xi, 122, 123
transparency, 78, 81, 84, 113
trauma, 122, 127, 133, 140
TRC, 2, 12, 15
treatment, 41, 42, 45, 48, 57, 70, 103, 113, 123, 126, 128, 139, 141
trial, 65, 118, 134, 141

V

vision, 48, 58, 77, 80, 86

W

Washington, 24, 60, 69, 114, 116
well-being, 39, 74, 81
workers, viii, 1, 8, 105
working conditions, 9, 10, 13, 15
worldwide, 30, 32, 43

Related Nova Publications

PUBLIC AND SCHOOL SAFETY: RISK ASSESSMENT, PERCEPTIONS AND MANAGEMENT STRATEGIES

EDITOR: Jarrett Conaway

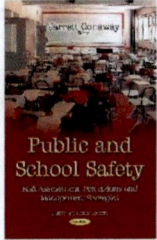

SERIES: Safety and Risk in Society

BOOK DESCRIPTION: This book discusses the EDURISC self-assessment questionnaire used for the assessment of integral safety in schools; provides insight on school indoor quality; and examines integration of chemical safety education into the preschool curriculum.

SOFTCOVER ISBN: 978-1-63117-223-6
RETAIL PRICE: $82

SAFETY CULTURE: PROGRESS, TRENDS AND CHALLENGES

EDITOR: Michel Sacré

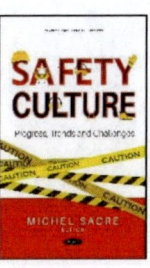

SERIES: Safety and Risk in Society

BOOK DESCRIPTION: In this compilation, the authors first analyze three components of safety culture: safety climate, safety values, and culture of prevention. The analysis includes both new empirical results and a review of earlier studies.

HARDCOVER ISBN: 978-1-53616-289-9
RETAIL PRICE: $230

To see a complete list of Nova publications, please visit our website at www.novapublishers.com

Related Nova Publications

OCCUPATIONAL STRESS: RISK FACTORS, PREVENTION AND MANAGEMENT STRATEGIES

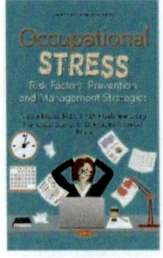

EDITORS: Nicola Mucci, MD, PhD, Gabriele Giorgi, PhD, Francesco Sderci, MD, and Giulio Arcangeli, MD

SERIES: Safety and Risk in Society

BOOK DESCRIPTION: Related work stress also generate significant costs, both direct and indirect, for companies. A budgeted economic investment will be use

HARDCOVER ISBN: 978-1-53615-404-7
RETAIL PRICE: $160

INDICATORS OF SCHOOL CRIME AND SAFETY

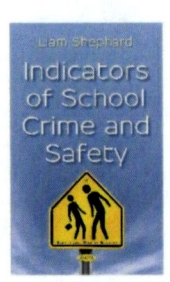

AUTHOR: Liam Shephard

SERIES: Safety and Risk in Society

BOOK DESCRIPTION: The report included in this book is the seventeenth in a series of annual publications produced jointly by the National Center for Education Statistics (NCES), Institute of Education Sciences (IES), in the U.S. Department of Education, and the Bureau of Justice Statistics (BJS) in the U.S. Department of Justice. This report presents the most recent data available on school crime and student safety.

HARDCOVER ISBN: 978-1-53613-680-7
RETAIL PRICE: $250

To see a complete list of Nova publications, please visit our website at www.novapublishers.com